LIVE YOUNGER, LIVE WISER

Pauline Noakes

BALBOA.
PRESS
A DIVISION OF HAY HOUSE

Balboa Press books may be ordered through booksellers or by contacting:

Balboa Press
A Division of Hay House
1663 Liberty Drive
Bloomington, IN 47403
www.balboapress.com
1 (877) 407-4847

Because of the dynamic nature of the Internet, any web addresses or links contained in this book may have changed since publication and may no longer be valid. The views expressed in this work are solely those of the author and do not necessarily reflect the views of the publisher, and the publisher hereby disclaims any responsibility for them.

The author of this book does not dispense medical advice or prescribe the use of any technique as a form of treatment for physical, emotional, or medical problems without the advice of a physician, either directly or indirectly. The intent of the author is only to offer information of a general nature to help you in your quest for emotional and spiritual well-being. In the event you use any of the information in this book for yourself, which is your constitutional right, the author and the publisher assume no responsibility for your actions.

Any people depicted in stock imagery provided by Thinkstock are models, and such images are being used for illustrative purposes only. Certain stock imagery © Thinkstock.

Print information available on the last page.

ISBN: 978-1-5043-8003-4 (sc)
ISBN: 978-1-5043-8004-1 (hc)
ISBN: 978-1-5043-8019-5 (e)

Library of Congress Control Number: 2017906841

Balboa Press rev. date: 06/06/2017

I wrote this book for people like me who seek to better understand the reasons for their health problems and who want to help themselves achieve optimal radiant wellbeing.

This book is not intended to deliver or replace medical advice.

Contents

INTRODUCTION

Why do we fall ill?

What makes it happen at all?

Is it bad luck?

Is life just plain unfair?

The question of why we become ill has been a major driving force in my life. I come from a family with a lot of health problems. We have osteoarthritis, cancer, asthma, eczema, thyroid problems, osteoporosis, heart disease, etc. etc. and my father wanted me to study medicine at university. The problem was that I did not want to do accident and emergency work, or surgery, or the procedures that I saw doctors having to do. As a teenager making choices about my career, that was what at that time I thought my daily work would be if I chose medicine. But I did want to know why one person developed cancer and another psoriasis; why did this one develop heart disease and that one arthritis? What made the difference? I needed to understand WHY.

Instead of medicine, I studied pure and applied mathematics, with physics as a subsidiary in the first year. My need for answers to my questions about the causes of health problems did not lessen and I spent hours with the medical students and psychology students that I knew, debating the issues. It seemed to me that medicine effectively and swiftly treated symptoms, but the same was not happening with cause. For anyone in a situation requiring Accident

& Emergency rapid-response assistance (following a road traffic accident or a bone fracture, for example), then modern medicine provided the best possible solutions and treatment. If, however, their problem was chronic and ongoing (such as heart disease or cancer or diabetes), then it was evidently not getting to the root of the problem.

In the treatment of chronic or long-term problems, a combination of approaches is needed to help manage the symptoms being experienced and to also find and address the cause of them. Some examples of this might be:

- Relief from physical pain (as in osteoarthritis, fibromyalgia, diverticulitis......)
- Reducing the limitations being placed upon the person's daily life by the condition (as in multiple sclerosis, rheumatoid arthritis, ulcerative colitis......)
- Alleviation of constant irritation and aggravation (as in eczema, tinnitus, allergic reactions......)
- Management of energy levels (as in chronic fatigue syndrome, hypothyroidism......).
- Healing body, mind and emotions (as in unhappiness, fear, depression, trauma.....)

In my search for answers to my questions over many years, I developed a serious set of health problems of my own and decided that I had to find answers that satisfied my cry of "WHY ME"? I had avidly read every nutrition magazine for many years, had a healthy diet and took some nutritional supplements based on the articles that I had read. I tried all manner of therapies in the UK and USA over a period of time and was still not finding anything that was making me feel better. I was still ill. Practitioner after practitioner (including medically trained doctors) told me that they could do nothing more for me as I was not responding to the treatment they were giving me. So, several thousands of pounds and dollars later, I decided that I had to find the answers I needed for myself.

Here's my story... ... ...

So there was I... ... . on a May evening in 1985... .... being told that I urgently needed tests and biopsies on two tumours that I didn't know I had.....!.

Well, that is some reality check.......!

I was working and living alone away from my homeland of the UK. The previous year, I had been offered a job in the USA and had decided that a complete change might be good for me....

I had put my house up for sale, given up my job, and moved three thousand miles across the planet to another country and a new life on my own. It was scary stuff and my dear parents were clearly more than upset that I was going, but did not try to tell me what I should or should not do with my life.

I made some good friends at the place I worked and, about a year after starting there, I asked a female friend what I should do about the routine cervical smear tests that all women were recommended to have. I had not needed to see a doctor of any kind since arriving there and, having grown up with the National Health Service in the UK, I was unsure about how the American healthcare system worked. I should add that I had no reason for having the test other than it had been a long time since I had had one.

I had had a severe eczema problem throughout my childhood and teenage years, but nothing else that I was aware of. I had been in bandages until I was sixteen years old. They covered my hands and arms, my feet and lower legs and other children would back away in horror as if I was the carrier of some dreadful disease that they might catch. The constant round-the-clock itching of the skin was a nightmare and I scratched and scratched until it bled, and then scratched some more. I would scratch between the layers of the bandages and the blood and weeping exudate would seep through the bandages and look like something out of a horror movie.

So my mother bought tubular gauze from the pharmacy and, for each arm, she sewed finger pockets in one end of the gauze to cover my hand and then pulled the gauze over the bandages up my arms, securing it with safety pins around the upper edge near the shoulder. So then, when I couldn't get between the layers of bandages to scratch, I would rub the area as hard as I could with my knuckles. I dreaded bath times because putting water on these areas intensified the constant torment of the itching and stinging.

My poor mother was desperate to try anything that would help. The family doctor prescribed what we called 'coal-tar ointment', a thick dark sticky substance that did nothing to stop the itching that was driving me crazy. In those days, bandages were washed and re-used and there was an old saucepan kept only for boiling my bandages. This was done on a daily basis and there were always bandages drying on a rack in the house.

Looking back on it now, I realise that I was a sick child but didn't comprehend that at the time. My skin problem was severe and obvious. I had little energy and everything was always "too much trouble". 'Life seemed like an unending series of struggles. "Oh, Mum, do I have to?" was my constant response to her telling me to get up in the morning or do anything that required much effort. In my teens, I was more often upright by willpower than by the exuberance of youth, as the fatigue was constant but unrecognised as a problem. I had always assumed that I was just a lazy child.

Anyhow…back to the smear test…. I decided to consult the local telephone directory to find a gynaecologist. I stopped at the first female entry that I found in the list and made an appointment with the lady. During my consultation with her at her office, she told me that her mother had had breast cancer, her sister had just had a mastectomy and that she, herself, had had seven biopsies in investigations for the presence of cancer in her own body.

She did the test for me and said she thought there was no problem. As was usual alongside the cervical smear test, she checked me for breast lumps and told me that I had a lump deep in the tissue on the right side. Lump? What lump?? I had had no idea that there was any kind of a problem. My beloved grandfather had died of cancer of the stomach when I was eighteen years of age, but I knew of no other incidence of the disease in the family on either side. And it had never crossed my mind that it might happen to me.

I was now in major panic. She said it was routine to check my blood pressure. This was certainly NOT a good time to be taking my blood pressure! And she was telling me that she wanted me to see her husband, a surgeon, for the next stage of attending to this lump that she had just found. I have no idea what I was saying to her in the terror rising inside me but, if anything could possibly make things worse than they already were in my opinion..... she then stopped in mid-sentence while still inflating the blood pressure monitor cuff on my arm, looked at my throat, and said "What's that lump in your throat?"

What... ... .????? It was 8pm on a Tuesday evening in May that I will never forget. I had thought that I was merely going for a routine health check and had no reason to suspect that any problem would be found. I had avidly studied everything I could find on nutrition since I was a teenager and my diet was good (I thought). I took nutritional supplements and I attended an aerobics class at least twice a week. I did not smoke. I had never used any recreational drugs, and the only alcohol that I drank was wine or the occasional Martini in social situations.

What a shock!! With such sudden unexpected bad news, the world seemed unreal. WHY ME? My brain could not process or compute what was happening to me. I looked at the doctor in alarm and said "What lump in my throat? She took my fingertips and placed them on the right side of my throat, just above the collarbone. "THAT lump", she said quietly. "That's not a lump", I argued. "I have glands in the throat that enlarge and shrink again at times but nothing that ever bothers me."

The doctor persisted with a barrage of questions. "Do you have problems breathing?" "What about swallowing?" "When was your throat last checked?"

What... ... .????? My throat had last been checked when I was six years old and surgery had followed to remove my tonsils. I had previously had surgery for the removal of my adenoids at the age of four years and any idea of being anaesthetised again after that for more procedures was nothing short of a total nightmare to me.

The doctor could not believe that I had not had a check in all those years and now was insisting that I see her husband, the surgeon. She said she wanted me to present myself at the local hospital at 8am the following morning (Wednesday) for blood tests. I could then go to work. On the second morning (Thursday) before going to work, I was to present myself again at the hospital at 8am for a mammogram to check the breast lump and to swallow radioactive pills in preparation for a scan of my throat. On the third morning (Friday) before going to work, I was to present myself once more at 8am for the scan of my throat.

I left her office in a daze. Living alone in a foreign country, no family or long-term friends around me, I was in turmoil. What on earth was going on? Why hadn't I known there was a problem? Was cancer so insidious that it was dangerously late before symptoms appeared? I had not reported any problem and here I was facing one of the most dreaded diagnoses of all. What had I done to deserve this?

My ability to sleep was then non-existent and I lay awake every night in constant panic, feeling completely out of control of my own body. I had been told that I had lumps, not only in breast, but also in throat, so what else might be going on that I couldn't see? Could I possibly have more lumps that I didn't know about in other places deep inside my body?

I had to keep going to work as normal. As employees, we had only two weeks and three 'personal' days for holiday each year. There was no time off for medical or other appointments. We were expected to take care of all that in our own time out of office hours.

The following week was like a whirlwind. I was working and then seeing doctors. I was adamant that I wanted a second opinion as I still couldn't take in the fact that I was really in this situation. I hoped to hear that there had been some terrible mistake. But… The next doctor that I saw to check the breast lump confirmed that there was indeed a lump deep in the tissue and he remarked on the thoroughness of the lady who had found it as it would not have been obvious to him. An urgent appointment was made for removal of the breast lump as the mammogram results were inconclusive. I was told that the probability was that the breast lump was malignant and the throat was not, so the breast needed to be attended to as the higher priority of the two areas of concern. And as soon as possible.

The week after the original visit to the gynaecologist, I walked into the operating theatre in a hospital gown in an oncology unit and put myself on the operating table. The surgeon wished me to have local anaesthesia rather than a general anaesthetic so that I would not need an overnight stay in hospital. My legs were strapped to the table, my right arm outstretched and, with no pre-med of any description to calm me, my stress levels were off the scale! I gripped the arm of the theatre nurse on my left side as if in a vice throughout the procedure and must have very nearly cut off the entire circulation of blood to her arm! My dentist later asked me what on earth I had been doing as my teeth looked like they had been subjected to some serious grinding…!

While I was still in the recovery room after the procedure, the surgeon popped his head around the door and said that the excised tissue had been checked by the laboratory and had proved to be non-malignant. He added that an appointment would be made in a couple of days to remove the drain that they had placed in the breast and then he left to have his lunch. Stage one done okay... ... Now what......?

Having a holiday was not an option and I had to keep working. Within a few days, I was at the office of an endocrinologist for the results of the throat scan. He showed no sign of urgency and, on realising that I was British, he recounted tales of his last trip to Europe. After a physical examination of my throat, he said that all the indications were that the lump in my throat was a "hot nodule" on the thyroid gland and so his advice was to "shut down" the action of the gland for a while to allow the nodule to shrink. If it did not shrink, then it would be wise to remove it surgically. I was given a prescription for thyroxin, a hormone produced by the thyroid, and told to return for a follow-up appointment three months later.

Although it sounded like I should be breathing a sigh of relief at this point, somehow that wasn't happening. The unease that I was feeling did not go away or lessen at all and I didn't know why. All I did know was that I was still totally bewildered by the series of events that had started on that Tuesday evening in the doctor's office. And I was still asking "Why me?" and none of the doctors had been able to give me an answer, other than shrugged shoulders and a look that said "That's life. You just have to get on with it!"

Shortly after starting the job in the USA, I had suffered a whiplash in a road traffic accident in which I was a passenger in the back of a van owned by the company that I worked for. There were no seat belts and I had been thrown across the back of the van by the impact of the collision with another vehicle. I had been a frequent visitor to a local chiropractor for treatments on my neck and back ever since the accident and so he now knew me quite well. I needed to continue with his treatment and, at each session, he listened to the latest update on my medical progress. When I told him about the "shutting down" of the thyroid, he looked horrified and recommended that I see a friend of his who was both a chiropractor and a kinesiologist. I had no idea what that was, but was feeling so unwell all the time that I was ready to try anything to feel better.

So off I went to see Kurt, the kinesiologist. He wasn't happy about "shutting down" the thyroid either, and he tested me for sensitivities to a long list of foods. The result of this was that I stopped eating foods containing gluten and/or milk and/or sugar. The first thing that showed improvement was the condition of my skin. I had never been a kid who wanted sweets and I usually gave away any chocolate given to me. But "stodge" was a completely different matter. I loved suet pudding, dry bread, pastry, anything made with flour. It was the texture that I liked. I also loved milk shakes and, in the health advice given for children at that point, our parents were told that milk was good for us. I loved anything made with milk -- custard, blancmange, bowls of cereal soaked in milk. The problems it could bring to asthma and eczema sufferers were not recognised back then.

Anyhow, back to my thyroid... ... ... I was on the diet without the aggravating foods, but my inner alarm bells were ringing louder and louder for no reason that I could find. There was just this rising panic going on inside me that nothing would subdue. I decided that I needed to come home to the UK, at least for a while, and then reconsider what I wanted to do when I was clearer about my health problems.

I went to see my family doctor in the UK with my X-rays and scan results and told him the whole story. He asked if a biopsy had been done on the nodule on the thyroid. When I said no, he wrote a referral for a consultation with a specialist surgeon at the nearest major hospital.

The day of the appointment at the hospital dawned some four months later, by which time I had a job working long hours on a big commercial IT project that was on tight deadlines and everybody was stressed! At least it distracted me from the constant worry about my health... ......

The surgeon extracted a tissue sample from the nodule on my thyroid into a syringe. As he checked the sample, the look on his face told me that my panic was well founded and that my inner alarm bells had been ringing for good reason all this time. He would not be drawn on a conclusion right there in his office but, within two days, I had received a letter from him confirming that the nodule was actually malignant and that urgent surgery had been arranged for four days later. I was told to present myself at the hospital for admission in three days' time.

I was now in a state of terror. My worst fear had been realised. I called him and asked if I could think about it. It was a bad time, from the point of view of project deadlines, to be missing from work. It was never going to be a good time, from my point of view, to undergo ANY surgery.

Was there any other way? Was there any possibility that the biopsy sample had been confused with somebody else's or that the diagnosis could be wrong? Was this some horrible drawn-out nightmare that I would wake from soon? The surgeon was short and sharp in his response, saying that there were several other patients needing that hospital bed and he would not have prioritised me for it if he had not deemed it to be urgent. He advised that I stopped asking questions and got myself in there without delay!

The thyroid is a gland shaped like a gentleman's bow-tie and it sits at the base of the throat. During the surgery, the entire right lobe of my thyroid was removed (that's where the tumour was) and also three-quarters of the left lobe ("just in case", I was told later). When this surgery is done, the next problem then becomes the parathyroids. These are four tiny glands attached to the extremities of the thyroid and they produce a hormone essential to the remodelling of bone.

Bone is a living matrix. Throughout our lives, mature bone tissue is being broken down and new bone tissue is being formed in the renewal process and also in the repair process (such as following a bone fracture, for instance). If the control of this process is disturbed, then osteoporosis can result. Some very skilled surgical work is needed to preserve the function of the parathyroid glands when thyroid tissue is removed. In the years since my almost-complete thyroidectomy, advances have been made in this type of surgery and it is now, I understand, much easier to do. I come from a family with a long history of osteoporosis and osteoarthritis and the last thing I needed, on top of my other problems, was complications in the bone department!

The doctors said they could do nothing further for me except follow-up checks over the next five years. My surgeon told me that the type of tumour that I had had can reappear somewhere in the body, typically in the breast or bone, up to fifty years later.

Not feeling particularly comforted, I set out to understand "Why me?" and realised that I had to find my own answers. I had been studying everything I could find, as well as attending courses, on nutrition for the past twenty years. I had implemented the recommendations on diet and nutritional supplementation. It had helped my general health a lot over those years but was clearly not the complete answer on its own. There was obviously much more to be done and I needed to find out what that was if I wanted to survive this. The search led me to giving up my job in the world of technology and retraining as a colonic hydrotherapist and then as a naturopath and kinesiologist and I found the passion of my life in alternative healthcare.

My journey has been life-changing, life-enhancing, difficult and glorious. It has provided me with reasons for why my health was the way it was. It has put the pieces in the jigsaw puzzle for me and given me answers that make sense. It has taken me on a route through the methods of modern medicine, through many complementary therapies and through training in the energy system of the human body and how it works.

For each of us, our health is our responsibility. We have to work at it. Without good health, life can become an endurance test instead of a joy. If we have a family history of life-threatening disease, or of conditions that reduce quality of life, we have to work even harder to overcome the risk of these same problems becoming manifested in our own lives.

Is preventive healthcare a part of your life? There are many things we can do to help ourselves and I hope with this book to give you some options that are easy to incorporate into your life to improve its quality. It will show you answers that I have found to my questions on this amazing journey. Except where stated otherwise, the opinions given are my own and the results of the conclusions I have reached. You may agree or disagree with them, but they put all the pieces of the puzzle in place and made sense of it all to me.

In this book, case histories have been used to illustrate the links between mental, emotional and physical problems. They are examples of how unresolved mental and emotional issues can affect the physical body and manifest chronic conditions. Names and identifying details of all those included in this text have been changed, but the impact of each person's experiences of health problems remain. By including them, I hope to help the reader interpret possibly longstanding issues on non-physical levels that are contributing relentlessly to persistent physical symptoms.

Along the way, I have been privileged to meet some inspirational people such as Dr Dietrich Klinghardt, MD, PhD, Richard Holding, DO, the late John Thie, DC, Professor Diana Mossop of the Institute of Phytobiophysics and the late Alan Sales of the Institute of Cyberkinetics and I thank them all for the inspiration and wisdom that they have shared with me. The wonderful skills of Kinesiology, originally developed by the late George Goodheart, DC, have enabled me to further investigate and arrive at answers for my questions.

So what IS it that makes a difference?"

Chapter 1

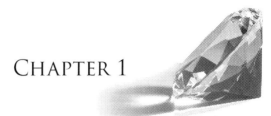

What exactly is disease?

How many of us worry about our health when we are young? Unless we have major health concerns of our own in our childhood years, or of someone dear to us, then we tend to think that we are invincible... ... ...

But, as the years advance, if we are challenged with health problems, whether those problems are big or small, our attitudes begin to change and we realise that ignoring them is not an option.

So, the question is, if you had known that you would live this long, would you have looked after yourself better?

How true is this for all of us? In modern day Western society in general, we don't want inconvenience, we don't want to have to make effort; we live in 'the disposable society'. We don't repair things; we throw them away. We expect everything to be instant and easy. We have computers, HD television, mobile phones and Wi-Fi.

We also expect our bodies to conform to this no-effort rule that we seem to have adopted. We know and accept that we have to maintain and service our car and put the appropriate fuel in the tank for it to work properly, but somehow we seem to have the idea that the same does not apply to our body, this vehicle that we live in during our earthly life.

We eat denatured and processed 'foods' that barely resemble real food. We eat and drink toxic chemicals and buy genetically modified foods. We live under huge mental and emotional stresses, such as those from family pressures, the need to pay the bills and meeting deadlines at work to keep our jobs. We often 'prop up' our lives with prescription or over-the-counter medications to keep us going. We need dental work from time to time, we are subject to scans, medical tests and procedures, vaccinations, the radiation from long-haul flights and airport security machines, the toxic air that we breathe, the impure water that we drink. And on and on.....

The brain is a bio-computer managing every function of the body via millions of electrical signals to and from every part of the body every second of our lives. These signals can be affected by other electrical fields around us. Thus, sitting in front of a computer all day, or using a mobile phone, for instance, can mean that "the captain is not properly in charge of the ship", by which I mean that the brain is not able to manage body processes effectively because its communications system is not able to function correctly in the presence of these fields in its environment. And, as more and more wireless technology is installed in our cities and workplaces, it is becoming impossible to avoid what Is sometimes termed "electrosmog", even if we choose not to install it within our own homes. As a result, we need to find a way of making our bodies more resilient to the sea of electromagnetic pollution that surrounds us but which we cannot see.

There is certainly a multitude of factors to consider in trying to find answers to chronic health issues. And how much can each one of us change things? Is it possible to reduce this electromagnetic pollution without affecting the lives that we have now grown used to? Have we thought about whether there could be a price tag on our health in order to maintain the modern-day life of instant results and ultra-convenience with our mobile phones and their internet capabilities available wherever we are, and with "smart" equipment in our homes?

Have you actually considered what your life may be like as you grow older? Or don't you want to think about it? Do you look at the older people in your community who have no control over their own lives because they can no longer cope on their own in any practical way -- and think that it won't happen to you? Do you think that your body should be able to keep going no matter how lax you are in looking after it? Do you put orange juice in your car tank instead of petrol or diesel and expect it to still operate as normal?

So where do we start with all this? Well, let's look at it pictorially. Imagine heaping all the well-known and acknowledged factors or stressors that can negatively affect your health and well-being into a pile. This pile would comprise items such as:

- processed foods;
- toxic chemicals such as formaldehyde and petrol fumes;
- toxic metals such as cadmium (from cigarette smoke or some paints) or mercury, nickel and silver (from amalgam fillings in your teeth);
- impure water;
- food additives such as aspartame (used as a sweetener);
- chemical sprays used in non-organic farming;
- bacteria and viruses;
- fungus and parasites;
- emotional trauma acquired in the school of life;
- and more and more.....

The size of this pile increases on a daily basis as more of these toxins pour into, and compromise, our systems.

Now imagine a wire fixed horizontally above the pile. While the top of the pile is way below the wire, the body is compensating adequately for the disruption that the toxins are causing and you will be thinking how lucky you are to be in good health. Your body will be finding 'work-arounds' for energy circuits that are not functioning correctly (by taking energy from other circuits, for example) to "keep the show on the road". The body is of such a phenomenal design that we are unaware of the compensations that it is constantly making every second of every day of our lives.

But, for all of us... when we fail to halt the advancing threats and onslaughts of the various stressors in our daily lives, and the day comes when the size of the pile has increased to the point where it now reaches the wire, we are in deep trouble as symptoms start to appear. It may be that we develop a skin problem, or symptoms of a bowel problem, or our thyroid function starts to wane or we start to develop the signs of a mental health problem or find a tumour somewhere or have a heart attack or stroke. Whatever the situation, the body cannot compensate adequately any longer and we need help.

The word disease breaks down into two syllables: dis-ease. The body is not at ease. Unbeknown to us, it has been battling relentlessly for a long time before we become aware of any problem. There have been imbalances occurring on an energetic level that a physical test would not have been able to determine or show. On the day that a heart attack occurs, for example, the imbalances in the energy system are now at such a level that the body cannot continue to "keep the show on the road" in any effective way any longer and the body is in need of urgent care and attention.

Consider the example of having a fire alarm on your house and the alarm bell keeps on sounding. Do you take down the fire alarm and throw it in the trash because it is annoying you by making all that noise, or do you investigate the fire that it is trying to tell you about?

Pain is like the fire alarm sounding. It is a warning to you that there is a problem somewhere in your body that needs attention. Swallowing analgesic medication to kill the pain is like throwing the fire alarm in the trash. The medication does not address the cause or source of the pain; it just stops the brain from feeling the pain. If you can't feel the pain, you may then think the problem has gone away, but the truth is that the "fire" is still raging and getting worse and you are now unaware of it. Does that sound like a great idea? The painkiller will only be effective for a short period of time and then the body will remind you again that it has a problem. Many people constantly take painkillers and do not address the reason for needing them. The body's struggle to achieve optimum health is already heavily compromised and this is now made harder by the additional load placed on it from taking the medication.

In terminal disease or after an accident, for example, medication offers unquestionably the best possible treatment. The comfort of the patient is the highest priority and the use of medication in palliative care is invaluable. In the case of chronic disease, however, medication can be essential in managing the situation but, all too often, the factors that are causing the symptoms are never investigated or treated.

The sad fact is that most of us become more and more dependent on medication as the years advance. We are in management mode, attempting to "keep the show on the road" as more and more problems develop and, in doing so, we add to the load on our bodies by introducing more drugs. Our bodies are unable to detoxify adequately and we get more toxic and more tired and more ill.

And, if we now acknowledge the added concerns of an energy system that is out of balance long before those symptoms ever appear at all, would we reconsider our definition of good health more carefully?

The increasing burden on the NHS is crippling it and the costs of running it are soaring. We need to find ways of helping ourselves so that we reduce the burden upon it and learn to take responsibility for our own health.

So what is YOUR definition of being healthy?

Do you describe good health as merely being without symptoms? Or is there more to it than that? I have heard people describe themselves as "fit and healthy" when they are walking with a stick and unable to lead a life independent of outside help! So is it all just a matter of expectations then... ......?

How about looking at the idea of good health as FREEDOM? Freedom to be active, freedom to make choices about what you would like to do today, freedom to walk, run, dance, stay in or go out. Without good health, these choices may not be available to you and there may be major restrictions on your lifestyle and therefore, also, major frustrations. Many would agree that, without our health, we have nothing, but we often only realise the truth of that when we, or someone dear to us, are/is confronted with serious health issues.

In the western world, we have grown up with a health system that allows us to hand over responsibility for our health to another person -- our doctor. We expect him or her to correct the problem for us, via drugs, injections and/or surgery. We do not usually see this as a team effort in which we should be playing a part. We don't like being told that our diet must change and our favourite foods must be eliminated or restricted. We don't like having to change our lifestyles. We generally don't want to hear that we have to do anything that involves effort or causes inconvenience to our lives. We want to do what we want to do when we want to do it and we don't want any consequences. So is what we really want the "magic wand" that fixes it all for us…?

Could we really make a difference to our health if we took some steps to change a few things? And, if so, what would those things have to be?

CHAPTER 2

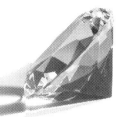

AM I LOOKING AFTER MY BODY WELL ENOUGH?

Trauma to the body can occur in many ways and not only on the physical level. It can also occur on the emotional and mental levels. Let us first look at the ways in which our bodies are frequently assaulted on a physical level.

We get one body for this lifetime and we may love it or hate it but we have to work with it. It may have health problems from the start (such as babies born with congenital defects) or it may develop problems later in life (due to infection or trauma, for example). And it may also have an elevated risk of developing some of the health conditions from which previous generations of the same family have suffered.

For the purpose of looking at physical damage to the body, it is useful to use the analogy of a motor car. If you consider your body to be a vehicle that you live in during your earthly life on this planet, you can make some comparisons with the way that you treat your motor car. If your motor car becomes damaged in some way (in a road traffic accident or by your negligence in maintaining it properly, for example), then you need to consider the level of the problem that results from this:

- Is it a write-off?
- Is it actually driveable at all?
- Is it safe to drive?
- Does it just need cosmetic repairs?

If your car is judged to be a write-off, is it truly beyond repair or is the cost of doing the extensive work that it now requires deemed to be just too great? How big is that cost exactly and does your desire to keep the car not make it worth it?

If your car is not driveable or not safe to drive in its current condition, then the damage has occurred in a crucial part of the engine or chassis. If so, the car cannot be used to transport you around without essential work being carried out by experts who are suitably trained and qualified to do such work. Without this work, the car will be unfit for its intended purpose and you will have to make a decision about whether you want the necessary work done.

If the level of damage is cosmetic, (say, there is a minor dent in a door or wing, but no damage to engine or chassis), then you can choose whether to address this in order that the car is "perfect" again or ignore it as it makes no difference to the running of the car and its use.

There is also, of course, the situation where there may be a part of the car not working correctly but the car appears to be running normally and you may be completely unaware of any problem. An example of this scenario may be the failure of a reversing light or brake light and, by continuing to drive the car in this condition, both car and driver are put at risk of major damage and the lives of others could also become affected.

Whatever the problem, how have you got here? How did your motor car get this way? Did you drive it recklessly, park it carelessly, fail to service it appropriately or forget to protect it adequately? Did you put water in its fuel tank instead of petrol or diesel and expect it to still do its job properly? Did you expect that it would reward you with years of loyal service if you neglected its needs?

If the damage to the car has occurred through no fault of your own (the dangerous driving of someone else, for example), you are still faced with the decisions about repairing it.

Now let's apply this analogy to your body, your personal vehicle for this lifetime. Do you think that your personal vehicle should keep on going no matter how you treat it? Do you become indignant, anxious, tearful and surprised when it grinds to a halt or tells you firmly that it can't go on any longer unless you make big changes to your lifestyle in order to consider its needs?

Sometimes it is essential that we have medical or dental interventions to save life or protect it. These may involve changing the body in some way from its original blueprint (removal of a gland or organ, for instance). We may need drugs or surgery at the hospital following an accident of some kind. Or we may need anaesthesia at the dentist's office to make the repair or extraction of a tooth more comfortable.

And by what other means could your body become changed from its original blueprint?

- Impacts (accidents or fights, for example)
- Sporting activities
- Cosmetic surgery
- Self-created trauma (tattoos are examples of this)
- Infections
- Toxic metals and chemicals
- Nutritional deficiencies
- Electromagnetic stress (such as radiation)
- As a result of emotional or mental trauma

How can you reduce this list?

Some of the answer to that question is self-evident. You may be somebody who loves sporting activities involving danger because it is exciting (an "adrenalin junkie") and so you know the risks that you are taking. Maybe you think that it won't happen to you anyway. Do you shrug your shoulders and say that you will have to take any consequences that result because your life is nothing without the thrills?

Excitement means different things to different people. Maybe you find the power of the mind more exciting -- new discoveries, advances in science, finding your unique creativity in the arts or music, perhaps. But these do not usually involve endangering the physical body .....

Unlike the motor car, your body is programmed to heal itself. We need to provide the nutrients that it needs to sustain life and to repair itself as necessary. This means looking at the fuel that we are "putting in the tank" (our dietary intake) and adding appropriate nutritional supplementation when the body is showing signs of struggle. In addition, we need to nourish it in other ways (such as clean air, pure water, adequate daylight, exercise and sleep) and protect it from any toxicity in its environment.

And the body will suffer if we do not attend to our needs on mental and emotional levels too. We need to be able to love and be loved. We need to be able to feel proud of our endeavours and achievements. We need to let go of our disappointments and dashed expectations instead of resenting them. We need to be able to find meaning in life's difficult challenges and to move forward with clarity and purpose.

So we could start by asking ourselves some questions:

- How often in my daily life am I actually focussed in the NOW? Am I typically trying to "fix" a past or future event in my life? In other words, (back to the analogy of the human body as a motor car), am I driving the car with my attention on the radio or on a discussion with a passenger in the car, rather than on the road and the traffic around me? Do I ever arrive at my destination with no memory of how I got there?

- Do I believe that I have any power in my own life? Am I proactive or reactive? Do I just wait for life to happen to me?
- How much do I really consider my true needs? Do I value myself enough or is my self-worth low?
- How big a price am I willing to pay, in terms of my health, in order to avoid taking responsibility for it?
- How can I help myself to heal the trauma and/or disease (if any) that has already happened?
- Do I believe that pain and suffering are an inevitable part of life? And, if so, is it possible to change that belief?
- Do I believe that a state of health, joy and well-being is actually achievable for me? And is there a way of making that happen within a life that is also exciting for me?
- Do I expect to live a long life that has quality right to the end?
- What is life really all about for me?

Stem cell researchers tell us that many of the cells of the body can renew themselves so that, at age 50, say, parts of your body are actually only around 10 years old (some of your bone tissues, for instance). Red blood cells can renew in 120 days and cells of the epidermis (surface skin cells) can renew in 2 weeks.

So, if you changed a few things in your life, could you possibly create a different body?

CHAPTER 3

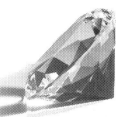

COULD I REALLY SLOW DOWN THE AGEING PROCESS?

Have you looked at the general health traits of the family into which you were born? Have you considered the patterns of disease in your ancestral lines or the conditions that have affected the members of both your mother's and your father's blood relatives? They can be a good indication of what might happen to you, as they show the possibility of increased risk of certain disease states.

In my own case, my mother was following in the footsteps of her own mother with crippling osteoarthritis, crying with the pain in her joints and starting to tell me that she was frightened because she couldn't remember things....

My father was so terrified of anything relating to the medical world that he would not tell anybody when he had pain or symptoms of any kind. He was completely phobic about injections, drugs and medical procedures and he would put up with any symptom in silence rather than admit to it for fear of what might be done to him. He believed that medical treatment meant him losing control over his life. And, because of this fear, he also did not want to know that anything might be wrong with my mother. She was the centre of his life, they had been together from their mid-teens at school and he could not cope without her. If she decided to have any kind of routine health check, she did not tell him as he would not have wanted her to go in case a problem was found. It may sound contradictory, but he always held the view that the ideal position with health problems was not to know. Then there would be no intervention and the body would put itself right, he thought. If there was a situation where the body did not put itself right, then there would be no option and it would have to be faced. But he didn't want to think about that…. In fact, he didn't want to go anywhere near a hospital at all, even as a visitor!

In my family, there was a history of asthma, eczema, thyroid problems, heart problems and cancer, in addition to the osteoporosis and osteoarthritis, so I needed to be paying attention… … … …

You may have a family history similar to mine. Are you doing as much as you can to take care of your body and keep yourself well in order to lower the risks of manifesting yet another case of any of the conditions frequently found in your family? We may be born into families that have high occurrences of, say, cardiovascular disease, or bone problems, or diabetes, for instance. As a specific example, if either of your parents have, or had, glaucoma (inappropriately raised pressures in the eyes), then the medical advice is to ensure that your own eyes are tested for this on a regular basis. If there is a family history of cancer or heart disease, then we are advised to undergo regular checks in order that any appearance of symptoms can be investigated and treated at an early stage.

Our ancestors were subject to diseases such as syphilis, gonorrhoea, tuberculosis and Bubonic plague. Survival is defined as the ability to adapt. Those who survived these diseases carried "imprints" in their energy systems as a result of their exposure to the disease. The human energy system is a multi-dimensional holographic network of energy pathways that intersect with universal energies around us. It contains a multitude of frequencies that may be discordant (imagine a mass of tangled hair and the tangles represent the "imprints"). Thus was created miasm, a disease taint which was then passed down the family line from one generation to the next. It may be seen as an "underlay" to chronic disease in this lifetime. Dr Samuel Hahnemann, the founder of homeopathy, was said to believe that miasm was "like a fog in the body".

These miasms affect the way that our energy systems can perform. As an example, if there is a high incidence of diabetes in the ancestral line, it does not mean that we will definitely develop it also, but it does mean that we need to take some sensible steps to help prevent it as our risk of developing the same disease may be raised. These steps may involve changing our regular diet to more health-inducing foods and making different choices about our lifestyle.

In the study of cell biology, it has been shown that our genes control the manufacture of biochemical substances in our cells. These substances make up, or further control, the structure of the human body. In other words, they make our bodies the way they are. But there are clearly countless differences in our bodies. We may have different coloured hair from our neighbour, or different coloured eyes or skin, and be heavier or slighter in frame, or be taller or shorter. And the list goes on.

Genes also affect the functions of the various systems, organs and glands of the human body. There are differences in the rate that some bodies age. Some people look much older than their years and some appear much younger. And, in addition, there are differences in the way that some of us react to certain foods, chemicals, drugs, etc.

These functional differences result from the way we "express" our genes, as they can send a different message under some circumstances than under others. So the decisions we make about how we live our lives on a daily basis affect whether we become ill or not because they affect the expression of our genes.

We have all seen the effect of extreme stress upon our friends and how it can alter their appearance, hair, complexion, etc. Similarly, we have also all seen the obvious results of a diet of fast foods, processed and/or sugar-laden foods containing little or no nutritional value. And the effect of long-term smoking or the use of recreational drugs upon the body is very evident.....

It has been shown in the work done by scientists in The Human Genome Project that changing our diet, the environment in which we live and work and our lifestyle choices, can all influence the expression of our genes and therefore influence the messages that they send. Thus the ways that you choose to eat and drink and run your life can change the way that your body ages and give you a more comfortable body to live in.

You may perhaps be carrying a gene that is known to make you more susceptible to a certain type of disease. The expression of that gene can be influenced by the choices that you make in your diet and lifestyle and how harmful your environment is to you

Or would you rather ignore the family history, live for today, decide that you will do what you want when you want and just hope that it doesn't happen to you? If so, and if you eventually find yourself in poor health as a result of not taking responsibility, what then? Have you considered the potential impact of your health problems, not only on your own life but also on the lives of those nearest and dearest to you? Do you have a vision of the future that assumes you will be in good health? Does the path to that vision include making the care of your health a priority?

As an example, you may have specific genes that make you sensitive to casein, the protein in milk. In this case, if you persist in consuming milk, you are likely to develop symptoms that may include swelling of lips or tongue, congested sinuses, ear infections, soreness in muscles and joints, irritable bowel syndrome, low energy, brain "fog", and redness and irritation of skin.

If your environment and/or lifestyle exposes you to toxic chemicals and/or metals, then you are more likely to develop disease if you cannot detoxify them effectively and quickly. For instance, if you are a smoker, or a taxi or bus driver (and so exposed continually to petrochemical fumes), or you live or work in a polluted environment, you may be at higher risk of breathing problems and respiratory disease. If, in addition, your diet consists of poor-quality foods, then your ability to detoxify adequately will be impaired and disease will result, possibly arthritis, depression or neurological problems.

Your genes themselves do not dictate the state of your health, but rather it is the ways that they express themselves that influence the way that your body ages. Thus you have more control over your health than you may think.

Perhaps the medical model of the future will be for doctors and health professionals to look at the risk factors for their patients and, in considering each individual's genetic differences, base their advice around reducing those factors with nutrient-rich foods and appropriate management of stress and attitude to life, as well as improving the environment in the home and the workplace.

We are all familiar with the foods that frequently cause problems to our health such as sugar and processed foods. They are well-known and widely publicised in newspaper and magazine articles about health and wellbeing. Information about healthy eating is easily and widely available to us.

The media regularly warns us all about the high cost of obesity to our health. There are literally hundreds of books on macrobiotic diets, vegan, vegetarian, high protein, raw food, low fat, low carbohydrate ways of eating, and none of us can honestly say that we were not aware of the foods that carry high risk of health problems, but many of us ignore all the warnings.

We often choose convenient, easy and low effort meals without regard to whether or not they contain additives and/or genetically modified foods and/or irradiated foods. We reach for fizzy drinks containing artificial sweeteners. We sacrifice our health for convenience and wonder why we end up toxic and tired. Lengthy periods of eating this way then, in turn, make us more likely to purchase more of these "convenience foods" because of the lack of effort required in preparing them and we no longer have much energy available for anything.

In an ideal world, a truly healthy person would be able to eat any food. The body would be able to assess that food effectively, and quickly and efficiently excrete it if the food is going to deplete the body's vital force. But, if the food is going to have a detrimental effect on your body and lower your energy levels, then why eat it at all? You are merely putting further stresses onto an already-stressed system as it now has to find the resources to get rid of the food again while gaining little or no benefit from it. Treating your body like a trash bin is no way of living younger!

If you are not eating sensibly and have let yourself get so hungry that you are ready to eat anything, then you are more likely to succumb to sugary snacks and drinks in an effort to pull yourself out of that energy dip that you now find yourself in. If this is your common state of being (i.e. tired all the time), then your body is showing you that your blood sugar needs better management. This means having an eating plan that nourishes your body and provides sufficient protein for your needs.

And continuing to consume sugary fizzy drinks may contribute to osteoporosis in later years, a condition where the bones deteriorate and lose their strength, and then mobility can become very limited. Is it worth it?

Ageing takes place when the cells of the body lose the ability to repair themselves. The captain is definitely not "in proper charge of the ship" and deterioration and dysfunction are progressing at a frightening rate and we feel powerless to stop them. But cells are intelligent and know how to repair themselves. So what has gone wrong? How did they lose their intelligence? How can we put the captain back in charge of the ship and reverse ageing into healing?

There's much more that we can do... ... ...

CHAPTER 4

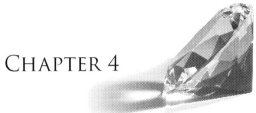

THE BOTTOM LINE.....

What happens when regular collections of rubbish do not take place in the area where you live? Do you see the rubbish piled up in the streets? Is that a healthy environment to live in? Have you seen the rubbish rotting when it is not removed promptly?

Do you think that there is a possibility that a similar scenario could be happening in your body? Does your personal rubbish get removed promptly and efficiently? Have you considered what might be happening in your body if not? If you do not get rid of your rubbish effectively, you will have an internal "compost heap" and you will not feel well.

In the story of my bid to regain my health following the discovery of cancer, I gave up my career in the world of computers to train in colonic hydrotherapy. I knew that I needed to make significant and big changes to my life if I was to survive this and I knew I was doing the right thing for me in changing career.

One person who thought it was a good decision was my friend Sharon, whose husband had died of bowel cancer the previous year at the age of 38 years. Simon had always been a fit healthy guy who had started complaining about episodes of what he thought was "indigestion" some months earlier. The discomfort had increased in both intensity and frequency and he was soon regularly taking packs of an over-the-counter product for indigestion. His wife implored him to go to the doctor but he repeatedly refused, saying that it was probably only a temporary situation that would soon go away.

When the packs of indigestion tablets that Simon was purchasing had reached ridiculous quantities and were clearly not solving the problem for him, he finally agreed to go to the doctor. He was referred to a consultant who decided to perform investigative surgery and, as a result, the surgeon pronounced that the tumour he found in the colon was inoperable and that nothing could be done. Simon passed away six months later.

Sharon encouraged me to take up the new career. She had witnessed the stress that I had been working under for so long, both personal (because of my health) and professional (because it was a high stress environment that I worked in). Maybe I was throwing away a good salary and years of training, but my life was at stake. A diagnosis of any kind of cancer prompts some rapid rethinking of what life is all about, and I had always wanted to work in alternative healthcare. So, if not now, then when …..?

There are many and varied problems that may occur in the processes of digestion and the elimination of waste from the body. In order to better understand what may cause those problems, we need to take a look at the work of the digestive system.

Your bowel is the last five feet of your very long gastrointestinal (GI) tract. Your GI tract is a hollow muscular tube which is open at both ends (mouth and anus) and the rest of your body is built around it (rather like a toilet roll). By the time the residue of the meal that you have just eaten reaches your bowel, it has travelled through your mouth, oesophagus, stomach and small intestine. So what has happened to it along the way?

The job of your teeth is to chop the food up as finely as possible so that you can get maximum nutritional benefit from it. You cannot extract the precious nutrients that your body needs if you swallow food in lumps and do not chew it thoroughly (so that means that eating "on the run" is not a good idea). You need to thoroughly mix the food with saliva to start to break it down in the mouth and also to lubricate the dry food so that it can move more easily through your digestive canal.

After you swallow it, the food moves down the oesophagus (a tube in your chest cavity that is about eleven inches long in an adult) into your stomach. There is a muscular partition (the diaphragm) between your chest cavity and your abdominal cavity and your stomach is a J-shaped organ lying just underneath the diaphragm on the left side. At the entrance to the stomach is a one-way valve to allow food into the stomach but not back the other way.

Since the stomach lies below the diaphragm, the lower part pf the oesophagus passes through a hole in the diaphragm and empties the swallowed food into the stomach. In some people, the hole in the diaphragm becomes stretched, the upper part of the stomach protrudes upwards through the stretched hole and the individual then has a condition known as hiatal hernia. This can cause great discomfort as acid reflux from the stomach can back up into the oesophagus, especially when the person is lying down or bending down.

The stomach acts as a temporary holding place for the food while it is mixed with gastric juice. This is a very acidic environment and should destroy any bacteria that may have been in the meal you have just eaten. The layers of muscle in the stomach walls create a churning movement to break apart the swallowed food and thoroughly mix it with the juice produced by glands in the stomach walls. Hydrochloric acid starts to break down the protein in the food (such as meat, fish or eggs) at this stage. It is evident, therefore, that if the body is not able to produce sufficient levels of hydrochloric acid or you are taking an antacid (acid suppressant), the proper breakdown of proteins in the stomach cannot take place and you will likely suffer from bloating and intestinal gas as a result (imagine rotting meat!).

When the liquefied food (called chyme) is ready to continue its journey onward from the stomach, the valve at the lower end of the stomach (known as the pyloric sphincter) opens and the chyme is squirted into the small intestine, a tube over fifteen feet in length in an adult. In the duodenum (the first section of this tube), the chyme is mixed with juices from the pancreas, the gall bladder and the glands of your small intestine wall. These juices break down the fats and carbohydrates in the food and complete the breakdown of the proteins before the chyme travels onward through the second and third sections of the small intestine (known as the jejunum and the ileum), propelled along by a process called peristalsis.

There are muscles in the intestinal walls that contract and relax in a rhythmical fashion, producing a wave-like motion to move the chyme along (much like the action of squeezing toothpaste from a tube). The ileum contains nodules of tissue called Peyer's Patches that provoke an immune response to any foreign substances from the environment (such as bacteria, for instance) that may have survived the acid in the stomach.

Most of the nutrients in the liquefied food are absorbed into your body in the long journey through your small intestine. There are lots of tiny projections and folds called villi (like fingers) on the internal walls of the small intestine that should assimilate the nutrients as the chyme passes through.

If you do not chew well and you swallow food in lumps, it is unlikely that it will be properly broken down. Unless the food is liquefied by the time it reaches the small intestine, its nutrients will be lost to the body because the villi will be unable to absorb them.

That means that you will derive little or no benefit from eating it. In fact, you will be using your much-needed energy to remove it from the body again and so you will have placed an unnecessary burden on your resources and wasted them.

In colon hydrotherapy sessions, undigested pieces of food (such as flakes of tuna and pieces of sweetcorn, for example) can be seen leaving the body whole when they have not been properly chewed and broken down.

After completing its journey through the small intestine, the remaining residue of the meal then passes into the large intestine (also known as the bowel or colon) through another one-way valve, called the ileo-caecal valve, at the lower right side of your abdomen. At this stage, the food residue should be like the consistency of thick soup. By the time it reaches the rectum (the final part of the bowel just above the anus), it needs to be in a formed stool to be expelled from your body in a muscular action. This means that most of the moisture must be absorbed into the body from the chyme during its journey travelling through the colon.

The large intestine is a tube around five feet long and two inches wide in an adult and it extends up the right side of your abdomen (known as the ascending colon), across the top just above your navel (the transverse colon) and down the left side (the descending colon), ending in the rectum and anus in the low centre.

At the lower end of the ascending colon is the caecum, a blind-end pouch from which your appendix hangs, in the lower right side of your abdomen. This is a popular place for some parasites to live if they have gained entry to the body (more of this later). The chyme must move upwards against gravity on the right side of the abdomen through the ascending colon to the level of the waist. At this point, the bowel turns left in a bend called the hepatic flexure just under the liver.

From the hepatic flexure, the food residue moves through the transverse colon across the body to a very steep bend called the splenic flexure on the left side at waist level. The transverse colon can sag or drop (prolapse) from the weight of matter left in there too long. If this happens, it can cause problems for the organs squashed below it (such as the uterus in females).

From the splenic flexure, the bowel bends sharply downwards on the left side (becoming the descending colon), ending in an S-shaped section called the sigmoid, which stops the now solid matter from passing too quickly into the rectum (the last part of the digestive tract, ending at the anus), where there are sphincters that help you control the expelling of faeces from the body.

The food residue is moved through your bowel by processes of peristalsis and mass movement, strong slow wave-like movements of the bowel walls that force the residue along. The bowel walls contain pockets, or pouches, which can expand or contract to accommodate large amounts of matter. Mucous is secreted by glands in the walls and this helps to move the food residue along whilst also protecting the walls themselves.

The digestive system needs energy to do its work. If we eat "on the run" or if we eat while upset or angry or while having an argument with someone (such as we see in movies where families constantly argue at the dinner table!), then most of the energy available is diverted to handle the emotional stress that is now going on, and so this energy is not available for digestion. The result is that the food is not broken down properly and we become bloated and uncomfortable.

Similarly, eating in a position where the torso is compressed (such as when watching television while sitting on a soft chair with a tray on the lap), the movement of the stomach while churning the food is restricted and the result is likely to be bloating and/or abdominal pain. The ideal situation for eating is in a calm tranquil environment, sitting on an upright chair at a table.

Food needs to be thoroughly chewed to almost liquefy it so that the saliva can do the best job. In order to produce enough saliva, we need to have food that looks attractive and smells good, in a variety of colours, on the plate. Then, when we chew, the saliva can mix thoroughly with the food and begin to break down the carbohydrates (bread, pastry, biscuits, beans, rice, for example).

During the years that I worked as a colon hydrotherapist, I heard some shocking stories from people who were struggling with bowels that did not work properly. Laxatives are one of the biggest selling over-the-counter drugs in the Western world and the subject of bowel function is not considered "nice" to discuss. Even in social situations, if people knew that I was doing colon hydrotherapy, they would come up to me and ask, in hushed voices, if they could please have some advice on their bowel problem.

During this time, I received a call from Amy, who told me that she was desperate. She said that she had not had a bowel movement for fifteen weeks. I asked her if she really meant that she had passed nothing at all in that period of time. She replied that this was indeed the case. When I questioned her further on the subject, she told me that poor bowel function had always been a problem for her throughout her life and that her usual pattern was that two weeks elapsed between successive bowel movements.

I pointed out to Amy that, in two weeks, she would have eaten forty-two meals, plus sundry snacks, and that one solitary bowel movement would not have effectively removed all the waste from that period of time! And that she should have sought medical help from her doctor a long time ago. Amy's response was that her doctor had prescribed the usual drugs available for chronic constipation over the years, but none of them had rectified the problem for her and so she had continued to struggle.

Amy proved to be not an isolated case, and I heard many similar stories of desperate people whose bowels did not function adequately and who consequently felt unwell and uncomfortable most of the time. In addition, there were others who had frequent diarrhoea and/or bowel urgency and were consequently afraid to go far from home because they always needed to be near a toilet, and so they felt that their lives were cruelly restricted as a result.

An example of the latter was Frances who was in on-going naturopathic kinesiology treatment with me. She had presented originally with pains in muscles of legs and hips, making movement difficult and very uncomfortable, and she also had a history of irritable bowel syndrome. Frances lived alone and had no family to help her and she was afraid that she might not be able to live independently for much longer. She had metals in her teeth in dental amalgam fillings that had been there for many years and, since starting her treatment with me, was in the process of gradually having the amalgam replaced with metal-free materials by a holistic dentist.

During one of her sessions with me at this time, Frances told me that her leg pain had reduced greatly and she was now able to do her shopping with ease but that she had been having diarrhoea, making her afraid to go out of the house for a different reason. She was taking the nutritional supplements that I had recommended for her and was making sure that she ate sufficient protein in her diet, but did not understand why her bowel was so problematic.

In my experience of practice over many years, kinesiology testing typically indicates a problem digesting corn and oats for anyone who has, or has had, amalgam fillings in his/her teeth. If all the amalgam has been removed and the mercury deposits trapped in the tissues of the body have been "mopped up" and excreted, then corn and oats typically no longer test negatively for that person. Upon testing in the same way, sugar and cow's milk are usually indicated as irritant foods for those with bowel problems, skin problems and/or asthma.

If these foods are excluded from the dietary intake, then this means avoiding most desserts and puddings, some cereals and biscuits, and some sauces (including those thickened with maize starch) unless some suitable replacement foods are found.

When diarrhoea is the problem, the body is attempting to remove aggravating foods as quickly as possible. In Frances' case, she had been so pleased that her muscular aches and pains had now gone that she had been regularly treating herself to her favourite desserts, thinking that her problems were behind her and that she could now eat whatever she liked without consequences. She wanted these foods and she was determined to have what she wanted! And her bowel was showing its objection by trying to get rid of them as fast as it could!

A few days later, she called me to confirm that her bowel problem had disappeared with the removal of the desserts from her diet and she was feeling happier and healthier as a result.

Frances was not an isolated case. Most of us are guilty at some time of eating foods that we know are likely to cause bloating, abdominal discomfort, bowel dysfunction and that sometimes also lead to obesity. Such foods frequently have little or no nutritional value and yet we eat them regularly as 'treats' to which we feel entitled. These foods are not treats for the body! If there is no nutritional value in a food, then you are using your body as a dustbin when you put it in your mouth. Your energy resources will be drained in trying to remove the offending foods again and you will be more toxic and more tired and also perhaps, as in Frances' case, in abdominal discomfort and unable to do what you want to do (i.e. go out and get on with your life).

This kind of scenario occurs each year in December as we celebrate the Christmas holidays. There are huge amounts of foods eaten as "treats" that have little or no nutritional value. It is no surprise, therefore, that the body "cleans house" every January and tries to rid itself of its rubbish any way it can. So it is common to develop coughs, congested sinuses, skin rashes, diarrhoea and to be low in energy at this time. Such symptoms are not necessarily indicative of a virus that is "being passed around" as is commonly believed... ... ...

Do you want a life where you live for now and never mind the consequences, or one that rewards you with radiant health and the ability to live a full and active life? Are you willing to do the work involved to achieve that?

CHAPTER 5

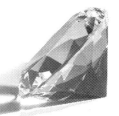

TOXINS? WHAT ARE THEY?

Toxins are organisms or substances that are harmful to the human body. They may originate outside the body and then gain entry into it (via food, for example). Some are produced within the body itself. They can become trapped in the tissues and cause irritation and inflammation that result in pain, discomfort, congestion and dysfunction.

Toxins that originate outside the body may be grouped into six main categories:

- Pathogenic bacteria
- Fungus
- Virus
- Parasites
- Chemicals
- Toxic metals

They may settle or accumulate in various parts of the body and proceed to adversely affect the function of the organ, gland or system in which they are trapped. This scenario therefore produces different symptoms depending on where the toxin is residing and exactly which toxin it is. For example, if the toxin is in the large intestine, the resulting symptoms may be those of irritable bowel syndrome, diverticulitis or colitis. In the joints, they may be those of osteoarthritis; in the brain, those of Alzheimer's or Parkinson's disease or multiple sclerosis, in the pancreas, those of diabetes, in the ears, those of tinnitus. And on and on .....

The many and varied diseases and chronic conditions with which mankind wrestles all involve the presence of toxins and modern medicine sometimes has no effective treatments to offer. Drugs may be available to reduce the symptoms and alleviate the discomfort or dysfunction, but they do not always address the root of the problem. The prolific use of some groups of antibiotic drugs in the treatment of bacteria has spawned its own new problem in creating drug-resistant species, resulting in a decrease in the effectiveness of these groups of drugs and generating a continuing kind of competition within the pharmaceutical agencies to find a solution.

Bacteria

Micro-organisms such as some bacteria or viruses, can live on the skin or in the body (in areas such as the intestine or mouth, for example) without causing disease. If the body does not have sufficient strength and resilience to defend itself adequately, some micro-organisms can invade it, leading to the development of disease.

In medical investigations for conditions where bacteria are suspected to be the primary causative agents, samples may be requested from urine, blood, sputum, faeces, cerebrospinal fluid and/or swabs from infected sites around the body. These samples enable the laboratory to isolate and identify the species that are relevant in each case.

Many species of bacteria are actually helpful, and sometimes essential, to our well-being (those that populate the intestinal tract, for example) and so the laboratory must isolate these bacteria from those that cause disease (known as pathogenic bacteria). The pathogenic bacteria can then be tested against a range of antibiotics to check which ones would provide the most effective therapy to eradicate them.

If the pathogenic organisms are difficult to isolate, then a blood sample may be tested. Whenever an infection occurs, the response of the immune system is to produce specific antibodies directed at the invading organisms. The blood sample is checked for rising amounts of these antibodies so that the appropriate medication can be prescribed.

The key to preventing infections is to support the body's defences and to maintain overall health so that the ability of pathogenic organisms to inhibit well-being in any way is severely limited and effectively undermined.

Fungus

The frequent use of some antibacterial drugs has created another set of problems for many people. The fungal condition commonly known as candida is the basis of a group of uncomfortable and distressing symptoms that may include:

- Thrush
- Fatigue and general weariness
- Skin rash
- Itching
- Excess mucus
- Constipation
- Diarrhoea
- Menstrual irregularities

- Mood swings
- Brain 'fog'
- Mouth ulcers
- Bloating
- Fungal patches on nails

We live with around 2kg in weight of bacteria in the intestinal tract and these bacteria have many jobs to do, including acting as "sentries" to control the presence of any fungus that may find its way there. These bacteria are sometimes referred to as the "friendly" bacteria in the gut. Antibacterial drugs inhibit bacterial growth and/or kill bacteria and infectious diseases such as streptococcus are successfully controlled by them.

After courses of some antibacterial drugs, the majority of the "friendly" bacteria are gone. The fungus is now uncontrolled and, in the presence of fermented carbohydrates and sugars (for example, a diet of biscuits, cakes, starchy foods and sweets), it proliferates rapidly and develops tendrils. Eventually, these tendrils can damage and irritate the wall of the intestinal tract.

Fungus is, however, usually a sign of a much bigger problem being present. Most of the symptoms that accompany fungus may also occur as a result of a viral infection. Fungus and virus can each produce chemicals that can cause unpleasant effects such as 'brain fog', inability to focus or concentrate, poor memory, skin irritation, inflammation, intestinal gas, mood swings and/or irritable bowel syndrome.

The fungus typically ceases to be a problem when toxic chemicals produced by virus are not active in the gut. If the presence of fungus is suspected following courses of antibiotics, then a good probiotic supplement will repopulate the gut with "friendly" bacteria. Otherwise, the virus usually needs to be the focus of attention for treatment.

Virus

Virus can cause inflammation of nerves, producing aches and pains and sometimes numbness or tingling via the toxic chemicals that it produces, and so it can be a factor in conditions such as arthritis, diverticulitis, fibromyalgia and colitis. It can contribute to congestion in the liver, reducing the body's ability to detoxify adequately. And then tiredness and a constant feeling of being unwell ensues (the "tired all the time" state of which so many people complain).

Some of the toxic waste from virus can confuse the immune system and prevent it being able to recognise the virus, thus ensuring that the virus can continue to thrive unhindered in the body. Some people may also develop allergic reactions to the substances produced by the virus.

And, as the liver becomes increasingly congested and sluggish, the digestive system starts to become affected too. The proper breakdown of proteins and fats becomes more difficult as the body struggles to produce adequate amounts of the hydrochloric acid and bile required to do this. Protein can then putrefy (rot) in the gut and bloating (and possibly constipation) may follow.

In conditions involving virus and/or fungus, it is important to avoid foods containing processed sugars (such as cakes, biscuits, sweets) as these foods feed both groups of toxins. Appropriate nutritional supplements can help improve liver function and digestion (and also deal with lack of energy if that is an issue too).

There are several herbal and homeopathic remedies that are helpful to combat the toxicity of virus in the body and to remove the chemicals produced by virus and fungus from the system. A qualified medical herbalist, homeopath or naturopath can help you find the remedies that will be most effective for you.

Parasites

Parasites can cause symptoms similar to those that result from candida and so it is important to get the right help to identify whether it is indeed parasites or candida at the root of the problem. In order to treat a parasitic infection, appropriate nutritional and herbal products can help relieve the symptoms, destroy the parasites and eliminate them from the body effectively.

Parasites are commonly described in two groups: protozoa and helminths.

- Protozoa are single celled organisms such as those that may be present in the urine of rats and mice.
- Helminths are worms and these are subdivided into three groups:
  - o nematodes: round worms that can vary in size from tiny threadworms to ascaris (several inches long)
  - o trematodes: flat worms such as liver fluke
  - o cestodes: tape worms that can grow to the length of the gastro-intestinal tract.

It is easy for parasites to gain access to your system. Some of the ways in which they may be picked up (if the sources are infected) include:

- Foreign travel
- Inadequate hygiene
- Improperly washed vegetables and fruit
- Drinking from cans
- Undercooked meat and fish
- Insect bites
- Supermarket trolley handles, door handles, light switches
- Money, telephones, computer keyboards

- Anything that has been handled by people who may not be washing their hands thoroughly enough.

Parasites are influenced by the energies of the full moon and some produce toxic substances that can enter the bloodstream and aggravate mucous membranes and thus it is possible that some symptoms caused by parasitic infection may be experienced as worse at these times. Again, a suitably qualified professional can help you determine which toxins are causing your symptoms and what remedies would be appropriate for you.

Chemicals

The body also has to deal with a constant barrage of chemical toxins which may include:

- Those that we ingest through our food (such as pesticides and herbicides that are sprayed onto many crops and vegetables, and also those fed to many animals, fish and birds that are then put into the food chain)
- Those that we inhale (petrol and diesel fumes and odours given off by some household cleaning products, for example)
- Those that enter our bodies through our skin (such as those present in some toiletries and cosmetics)
- Those from long-term use of some drugs
- Those that are present in our immediate daily environment at work and home (glues, plastics, solvents, paints, furniture and fabric finishes, for example).

If your detoxification system is unable to cope, you may become hypersensitive to environmental chemicals and experience symptoms such as:

- Fatigue, lethargy, exhaustion
- Impaired memory and/or concentration
- Confusion, "brain fog"
- Panic attacks, irritability, restlessness
- Headaches, insomnia
- Depression
- Co-ordination and/or balance problems
- Numbness, tingling
- Behaviour/personality changes
- Aches, pains, weakness in muscles
- Nausea, abdominal pain/cramp
- Bowel disturbances
- Blurred vision, conjunctivitis
- Laryngitis, sore throat
- Food allergies, intolerances

Toxins daily find their way into the body from the outside. In addition to these, there are other toxins produced by any organisms that have previously gained access to the inside (virus, for instance). And, to add even more to this load, we also produce other toxins ourselves within the body as by-products of biochemical processes that are taking place all the time.

Toxic metals

If we are feeling unwell over a period of a few hours and there is no obvious reason for our current pain or discomfort (so not resulting from an accident of some kind, for example), then we might initially question what we have eaten or drunk recently that could be responsible for our malaise.

If the situation persists beyond being a temporary problem and becomes an on-going one, we consider the possibility of an infection. The body can find itself under attack from sources such as bacteria, virus, an insect bite or the ingestion of parasites or their eggs. It can also be reacting to the ingestion of toxic chemicals.

If the condition becomes chronic, there may be an additional factor contributing to the dis-ease of the body, that of toxic metals.

Bacteria, viruses and parasites are well known contributors to disease and vast amounts of money are continually spent on researching their effects on the body and on finding effective drugs to combat them.

But waging a war on a variety of organisms is a very different scenario to addressing the problems caused by toxic metals in the body. The obvious and most major difference is that metals are not living organisms, and so the removal of metals cannot be approached in the same way.

Many of us have no idea that we have toxic metals in our systems and, indeed, how they might get in there at all. Some of these metals have been associated with symptoms that have proved difficult to treat and modern medicine to date offers no drugs that are effective in removing them from the body and therefore can only alleviate the symptoms for the patient with the use of drugs (painkillers or steroids, for example).

Levels of toxic metals build up in the body over a period of time and early symptoms may be slight, graduating over time to more severe warnings (such as memory loss or abdominal pain, for instance). If we want to live younger, we need to pay attention to finding a way of clearing these metals.

Many of us are hypersensitive to some of these metals, making their adverse effects on the body even greater. They may affect the nervous system, the immune system, the hormones, the digestive system, the kidneys, brain and heart.

So what are these metals and how do they get into the body? The following paragraphs take a look at the most common ones.

- Mercury

  The most common point of entry of mercury into the human body is by the use of dental amalgam for fillings in the teeth. Dental amalgam is a combination of several metals (typically mercury, silver, tin and copper), of which mercury is the primary constituent.

  Amalgam has been used in dentistry for decades because of its low cost and high resilience. Mercury can be a factor in pain, inflammation and congestion in body tissues. It can adversely affect hormonal pathways and cause dysfunction of organs and glands. Its use in dentistry has been restricted in some countries and it is not permitted for use in dental work for pregnant women in some others. It has been used in a preservative (called thimerosal) in some vaccines.

  Symptoms such as back pain, headaches, insomnia, tremors, mood swings, chronic fatigue, muscle weakness and more have all been associated with the presence of mercury in the body.

  Toxic metals can be discharged from pregnant women to their babies in the womb via the placenta and, after birth, via breast milk. Including the removal of toxic metals as part of preconceptual care where possible can help both mother and child.

  Increasing numbers of dentists are recognising the long-term problems that can be caused by placing toxic metals into the mouth in dental procedures. Many new metal-free materials that are suitable for use in dentistry have been developed over the past few years and it is now easy to find a dental practice that advertises metal-free work. Some people have dental crowns or onlays that have been placed over teeth that contain dental amalgam and so these may need investigation as well.

Those dentists who recognise the possible detrimental effects on health of toxic metal used in dentistry usually adopt a cautious approach to the removal of the metal, with great attention to methods of protecting the patient from ingesting the metal as it is drilled out.

Ask your dentist about the barriers that he or she intends to use when removing metal from your teeth and also about the materials that will be used to replace it. Alongside the dentistry, a program of appropriate nutritional supplements would support the "mopping up" of the toxic metals and assist the body in excreting them efficiently.

- Lead
  For many years, lead was introduced to the body via the use of lead pipes to deliver water to homes and offices, from the use of leaded petrol and certain paints and alloys. So, from the days of fumes from leaded petrol, for instance, if you spent time cycling in traffic without a mask, or lots of time driving, or if you lived in the city and walked a lot, you may have ingested lead into your system. It has been linked to symptoms of fatigue, irritability, tremors, memory loss, insomnia, infertility, constipation and more…

- Aluminium
  Aluminium is present in many household items, from some types of cookware to some brands of toothpaste. Aluminium salts may be used to block the pores in anti-perspirant products. In the form of "tin foil", aluminium

is used in many kitchens for cooking and storing food. Its presence in body tissues has been linked to symptoms of loss of co-ordination, loss of memory, confusion, osteoporosis, lymphatic congestion and more...

- Cadmium
  A common source of cadmium in the body is cigarette smoke, and it is also present in some paints and alloys. Many of us have smoked or lived with smokers. Even if we ourselves have never smoked, we may have spent lots of time in bars and restaurants inhaling the smoke of others during the years that it was permitted in public places. Cadmium has been linked to symptoms of aches and pains in muscles and joints, skin problems, fatigue, mood swings and more...

Toxic metals may be released during some industrial processes and be present in the air that we breathe and the water that we drink. In some areas, the drinking water may sometimes taste 'metallic' and it is possible to filter the water you use for drinking and cooking and also the water you use for bathing. And concerns have been raised about the possible toxic effect of energy-saving light bulbs as they contain some mercury and need to be disposed of very carefully.

If you used to smoke, but no longer do, then are you thinking that cadmium is not a problem for you? People typically assume that, if they are no longer exposed to the particular metal (for example, in the instance of having given up smoking), then that metal cannot now be a problem for them and cannot be a factor in their symptoms.

Whatever way you may have ingested any toxic metal at any time in your life, your body will try to protect itself from it by "locking it out of the way" for safety. So where would be useful for this? Energy testing methods (as used in kinesiology, for instance) have linked the presence of toxic metals to sites in the brain, thyroid, kidneys, bladder, pancreas, the lining of your digestive tract, your joints, and more ... ... Other methods are also available for testing for the presence of toxic metals in the body (hair analysis, for example). In the body, fats make an easy place to lock away toxins and we have trillions of cells with lipid (fats) membranes. And toxic metal has also been found to be a contributing factor in the greying of hair as we get older.

Tattoos have become a popular way of decorating the human body in recent years. Health warnings have been raised about the possibility of bacterial contamination of the inks injected into the skin. Little has been said about the toxic metals that are used to produce the colours of the ink. So could tattoos elevate the risks of health problems in the future?

Should we be paying more attention to the inside of the body than the outside? Doesn't the condition of the outside of the body follow how we look after the inside of it?

The role of the liver in detoxification

Imagine the body as a factory and, inside this factory, there is a conveyor belt carrying a never-ending huge load of toxic materials towards, and into, a machine (the liver) that will turn these materials into safer forms that will no longer be able to poison their environment and cause damage. As they leave the machine, these safer forms are then loaded onto other conveyor belts that take them through exit routes and out of the factory completely (this would be through the bowel, for instance).

You can then see the way that many of the problems that contribute to disease arise when you consider:

- What if the machine is clogged up and too congested to take any more input?
- What if it is inefficient because it does not have enough of the appropriate fuel to do the job properly?
- What if some of the toxic materials are still toxic when they leave the machine because the machine is not being maintained sufficiently well?
- What damage will these unprocessed and still-poisonous materials do to their environment inside the factory before they reach the exits?
- What if any of the exit routes are jammed and backing up and the still-toxic materials coming out of the machine are now spilling over into other parts of the factory and causing damage there?
- What if the machine has been so abused and neglected over time that it can't do the job effectively any longer and the situation within the factory is now out of control?
- How can other departments of the factory do their jobs when they are damaged and overloaded and more and more of these toxic materials are arriving every day?

This scenario paints the picture of why it is vitally important for all of us to have a body that can clean itself effectively and efficiently. Proper care of the liver is central to that need and the liver must be given the essential nutrients that it needs to do the job. If those nutrients are not there, then other organs, glands and systems begin to suffer as the overflow of toxic waste poisons them. Then we are told that our blood sugar is too high, our cholesterol is too high, our joints are deteriorating, our heart is under strain, we are becoming diabetic, and on and on... ... ...

We can help ourselves to stay healthy in many ways. But what if we find a lump somewhere....? Doctors tell us to check ourselves routinely for lumps and to report any instances of bleeding from bladder or bowel as they may be symptoms of malignancy. If caught early, medical treatment can undoubtedly prolong lives by removing the tumour.

But is the tumour itself the cause of the problem or is it the result of other underlying factors? The removal of the tumour may be an urgent necessity, particularly if the tumour is blocking a major route such as the airway or the bowel, for instance. But is that the end of the problem?

There must have been some kind of energy that caused that tumour to grow and to proliferate and which is still present in the body's system and able to "set up home" in some other tissue. Thus the scenario of recurrence always looms threateningly for the cancer patient and some of them resort to further surgery, with all that that implies in pain, stress, loss of working time, etc., "just in case".

Living in constant fear is not a pleasant place to be and contributes to diminishing immune function and the body's waning ability to withstand the pressures of everyday life. Anyone who has had cancer dreads the follow-up appointments and health checks in case they are told that the cancer has returned or spread.

For those of us that have a diagnosis of diabetes or arthritis or any other chronic condition, how can we reduce the load on our already-overburdened medical services, help ourselves to feel better about our lives and to be more able to keep ourselves well?

Medical science has created specialties of focus and expertise in the different areas of medicine. If we have a problem in the digestive system, we go to the gastroenterologist. If we have a heart problem, we go to the cardiologist. If we have a hormonal problem, we go to the endocrinologist. If we have a skin problem, we go to the dermatologist. Health problems are addressed within the discipline indicated by the signs and symptoms.

In the holistic approach to chronic disease (as used in therapies such as naturopathy, for instance), the body is addressed as one whole system in which everything affects everything. When it is threatened by infection or other circumstance, the response of the body is to try to recover its optimal steady state of equilibrium, excreting the toxins efficiently, restoring normal function, repairing damaged tissue and generating new tissue where necessary. Holistic therapies support these processes by a combination of natural remedies that may include nutrition, herbs, homeopathy, energy work (as in acupuncture and kinesiology, for example), counselling and meditation.

In the 21st century, we live in a toxic environment and we inevitably ingest toxins into our systems. Wherever the toxins are trapped in the body, the function of that particular organ, system, gland or tissue is negatively affected. Thus it cannot do its job properly and we accordingly experience symptoms linked to that dysfunction. In some cases, this may, in turn, lead to dis-ease elsewhere in the body and so the source of the current complaint is not always where we expect it to be.

The same toxins can be responsible, directly and indirectly, for a huge array of different symptoms in the body. The following chapter considers factors that influence where the toxins will trap in the body for each individual person. It looks at how the state of our own physical body can indicate the extent to which we have avoided sorting our emotional and mental "stuff"! This is a simplistic model of a multiplicity of complex problems, but it seems to answer most of the questions that are commonly asked.

Both medical science and holistic therapies have much to offer in the treatment of chronic disease and integrated methods can remedy:

- Physical discomfort and dysfunction (e.g. relief of pain, reduction of inflammation)
- Torment and unhappiness (pain on emotional and mental levels) in order to allow the trapped toxins to be eliminated from the body
- The harmful effects of the environment that disturb the energy matrix of the human body and that disrupt its internal communications system.
- The resources that the body needs to repair and regenerate its cells and tissues.

Can we feel less power<u>less</u> and more power<u>ful</u> in such a situation? Can we rid ourselves of the toxins and toxic substances that have accumulated in our bodies over the years and, in order to do that, shouldn't we be addressing the mental and emotional factors that have allowed the toxins to become trapped in the tissues?

CHAPTER 6

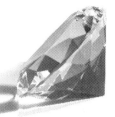

LIFE'S LESSONS

Your body is made up of trillions of cells. The cells have a memory and they transmit information to each other.

But are you only your body? Do you identify yourself with just your physical body or do you think that it is possible that some other part of you could exist on some other unseen level too?

You have an energy system driving the physical body, directing the repair and renewal of its cells via a field of information that "keeps the show on the road", so to speak. So is it possible to influence this energy system in any way and, in doing so, also influence the biological ageing of your body?

I was always fascinated by what makes people "tick". Why do some people react so differently from others when facing the same situation? If the situation is a painful one, some of us seem to be able to pick ourselves up, find a new focus in our lives and move on beyond the experience. Others may be completely unable to cope and may sink into depression, or become aggressive or cynical perhaps.

We learn and grow in this lifetime through the ways that we handle the challenges that life brings to us. We react instinctively according to patterns in our psyche. In astrological psychology, the way you instinctively react as an individual is indicated by the position of the Moon in your natal chart. So, for instance, with Moon in Taurus, when faced with a difficult situation, you would tend to react with stubbornness, dig your heels in and want to deal with it in the way that you always have, thus resisting change or being taken out of your comfort zone in any way.

Emotional and mental trauma, if ignored and/or not given the help and attention that it needs to resolve it appropriately, manifests as physical dis-ease in the body. The symptoms that develop are the body's way of telling us where and what we need to heal.

As we go through the school of life, we are presented with many challenges and many opportunities, but we often don't see them as that (and sometimes we don't see them at all!). If we suppress or internalise trauma on emotional and mental levels, the body's only way of showing us that it needs help is by the appearance of signs and/or symptoms. It shows us physically that it is in distress so that we can see or feel that there is a problem (by the onset of pain or the appearance of a skin rash, for example). If the symptoms are not severe, we may choose to ignore them for a while but, eventually, ignoring them will no longer be an option. The underlay for chronic disease is in place.

Some of the challenges that may face us in the school of life may leave us feeling totally powerless and in despair. At some point, it is likely that we will experience the heartache and helplessness of bereavement when a much-loved parent, partner, family member, friend or pet dies. Some of us may experience the pain of rejection or abandonment if a partner leaves us for another, or a parent decides to leave the family home. The deep wounds that these, and other hugely painful events, leave on our lives can feel like a permanent form of torture. If they happen in our childhood years, such wounds can run particularly deep and we usually learn to develop survival mechanisms for self-protection, which may involve withdrawal or behavioural problems or attention-seeking ploys.

Many of us permanently carry resentment and bitterness that life has been unfair to us and we feel powerless to do anything about it. Living this way results in a "helpless and hopeless" state, often referred to as a "victim" state, in which we tend to look for someone or something to blame. This may be expressed in opinions such as "I was never good enough – my brother was always the favourite child" or "It was my father's fault – he left home when I was young and showed no interest in me" or in any of a multitude of variations on the injustices that we feel have inflicted pain upon our lives and that are ultimately responsible for our unhappiness.

In this state, we may withdraw, put up our barriers and seethe and fester with resentment inside, or we may try to seal off the pain somehow and pretend that we're okay – but we fool no-one! The pain shows in our attitude (and ultimately in our faces) in the way that we present ourselves to the outside world and in our insistence that nothing is wrong when that is obviously not the case.

Others of us may respond to unbearable emotional pain by becoming needy. It may feel like we have an empty void inside that nothing can ever fill and that we will never be able to find appropriate comfort. In some cases, we may turn to substances such as drugs or alcohol to numb the anguish that we feel. Or we may become self-indulgent, turning to excessive amounts of food for comfort, especially chocolate or other sweet or stodgy foods. Some of us become bulimic and repeatedly throw up the food again in our efforts to prevent the usual results of eating binges (weight gain, bloating, bowel problems, flatulence, fatigue, etc.). Some bulimia sufferers have spoken of their accompanying release of anger and rage towards "what life has done to me" when they throw up.

Without the appropriate help for our distress, our bodies can pay a high price for the continual pressure of the trauma, and we may also unintentionally bring pain to the lives of those around us. The price that we pay may include physical pain, restriction of movement and loss or disturbance of function. As a result of the scars and wounds that remain unhealed, we may experience increasing levels of back and/or muscle pain, for example, as the body shows us its desperation for help on a non-physical level.

We may be constantly held back from taking opportunities in life because of fear. Fears that are commonly expressed include:

- Fear of failure
- Fear of success
- Fear of expressing our true feelings
- Fear of being judged by others
- Fear of change
- Fear of loss
- Fear of pain
- Fear of being alone
- Fear of intimacy
- Fear of shame
- Fear of not having "enough"
- Fear of fear itself
- Fear of commitment
- Fear of the unknown

As we go through the school of life, we experience many emotions as we react to the opportunities and challenges presented to us. Each different emotion has its own energetic frequency. Each different type of body tissue has its own energetic frequency. Negative emotions (such as fear, anger, guilt or rage, for example) restrict the proper functions of the parts of the body with similar energetic frequencies and allow toxins to become trapped there, paving the way for symptoms such as physical pain and inflammation to develop. The physical follows the emotional.

The body shows us, in developing a physical problem, what the emotional problem is and therefore what we need to address in our lives.

To illustrate what this means, we can look at emotional factors that contribute to some common health problems, starting with perhaps the most common complaint of all.

The power of seeing the world without anger

Toxic and tired?

Many of us complain of being "tired all the time". A primary consideration in such a situation is how the liver is functioning. Among its many different jobs, the liver is central to the ability of the body to remove the toxins that are ingested into it on a daily basis via the mouth (in the foods, drinks and, possibly, some drugs that we consume), the lungs (in the air that we breathe) and the skin (in the substances that we put into and onto it). If the liver is not able to do the job properly, one of the results is that we can become toxic and tired.

But why wouldn't it be able to do the job properly? We can look for organisms or toxic metals (virus or mercury, for example) that can inhibit proper function of the liver. We can also look for deficiencies of the nutrients that the liver needs to do its work (the "fuel for the boiler", so to speak). But will checking all the possible contributing factors on the physical level provide the whole story?

In order to see the true picture of the burden under which the liver is struggling, we also need to consider the emotions and, in particular, the issue of anger. Some of us seem to spend our lives being angry. Some of us say that others comment that we seem angry and we really have no idea what they are talking about. We may find ourselves repeatedly justifying our right to be angry. We may be carrying anger towards a family member, an ex-partner, a former friend whom we perceive as having let us down in some way or, perhaps, towards bullies at school or at work, whether past or present. We may find it difficult to actually acknowledge our anger.

While we continue to be angry for whatever reason, our physical body is paying a high price. The impact of anger is felt in the liver. When we persist in being angry, we are compromising its ability to function efficiently and, since the liver performs a multitude of functions in the body, the resulting symptoms may be many and varied (hormonal imbalances or a sluggish colon, for instance). And, if toxic and tired is our usual state of being, the issue of anger may be a key factor.

The power of seeing the world without rage

Some of us regularly storm around in a rage, feeling like our temper is out of control. We often describe things that "make our blood boil". We may be accused of being aggressive to others or in our attitude to life. Until we resolve the cause(s) of the rage and find some calmness and tranquillity in our lives, the function of our gallbladder may be impaired.

The gallbladder sits next to the liver on the right side of the body, just above waist level, and stores the bile produced by the liver, releasing it into the small intestine as and when required to help with the digestion of fats. The release of the bile is controlled by a valve in the biliary tract called the sphincter of Oddi and this valve may become dysfunctional in people with unresolved issues of rage. When this occurs, the flow of bile may not be adequate to meet the need for it and so there may be phases of problems digesting fatty foods. Bile is also the substance that gives colour to the faecal matter, so if you are expelling pale or sandy-coloured stools from the bowel, then the supply of bile by the liver and gallbladder may need attention (and, very likely, so does your level of anger and rage).

The power of seeing the world in
the present, not the past

In our physical body, the bowel represents letting go of the past and ridding ourselves of the rubbish that we no longer need. The physical follows the emotional and so we need to look at what "rubbish" we may be holding on to on the emotional level if we have a bowel problem. This "rubbish" may be guilt and remorse resulting from "bad" decisions and/or behaviours on our part that caused pain to ourselves and to others.

If there is something in the past that we constantly wish that we had, or had not, done or said, we feel that we are powerless to "fix" it and that we are being punished by that particular record going around and around in our head. Living in, or holding on to, the past can cause us to miss opportunities that life is offering us in the present.

Past events that are continuing to cause us pain can teach us lessons about becoming a more compassionate person in the future and about making choices and decisions in a wiser way from here on. But if we live in the past, without learning anything from it, just constantly going over and over situations that happened previously, we feel more helpless and more powerless and we hold onto our "rubbish" and prevent ourselves from moving on with our lives. Thus, the rubbish piles up in emotional terms and the physical body reflects that situation in a problematic bowel.

So while we are holding on to the guilt and remorse, the bowel is holding on to the waste matter too. The main job of the bowel is to excrete the stuff that the body has decided it doesn't need. At the end of the processes to digest our food (and hopefully get some nourishment from it), the bowel should excrete the waste, along with other residues from the repair and regeneration processes that have been going on all the time in the tissues. There is no benefit to the body of holding on to any of that!

Such a situation may manifest as constipation, diarrhoea, colitis, diverticulitis, or be called irritable bowel syndrome or inflammatory bowel disease. And, it's not only the physical body that may show the strain. Recurrent bad dreams and/or phobias may become a problem too.

It is no surprise to find that an untreated bowel problem next progresses to a problem in the liver, where we hold our anger (and we may be angry with ourselves and/or with life in general).

We can help ourselves the most by making a decision to change, from here on, the behaviours and/or ways of thinking that have caused us so much pain. If we don't learn from them, then we have missed a big lesson and an opportunity to change our future and improve our health hugely.

The power of seeing the world without bitterness or resentment

When we constantly compare our lives to the lives of others and only see what is "better" in theirs, we affirm to ourselves that "Life is not fair" and that these others have an easier time than we do. We are putting ourselves in a place of lack, of never being able to have what "they" have and expecting that life will always be this way for us.

In this mode of thinking, we are in a victim state. We feel powerless, believing that life "happens to us", that it is completely beyond our control and that having the ability to change it is an impossible dream.

In victim mode, we typically find it difficult to forgive. We may express our feelings with sarcasm. We often have a tendency to withdraw emotionally from people to "spite" them. And we may be taking it out on ourselves too by treating ourselves badly in some way (smoking or not eating sensibly, for example).

If there is someone whom we need to forgive, then is there a different way that we could look at the particular situation with this person/company/organisation that enables us to be kinder to ourselves and let go of the bitterness that we are holding? Haven't we already suffered enough because of this issue? Whom does it serve that we continue to suffer? Isn't it limiting our life and our enjoyment of it by reminding us of unhappy times? How big a price are we willing to pay in order to justify our position and be right?

Do we need to forgive ourselves for things that we have done or said? Do we constantly berate ourselves for having been "stupid" or "weak" in some situation(s)? Is "I shouldn't have done that!" running over and over in our thoughts? Or "I hate myself for being so stupid (or so weak)"?

Harbouring resentment and bitterness may be contributing to lung problems such as chronic obstructive pulmonary disease (COPD), emphysema, pleurisy and asthma. In some instances, they may contribute to osteoporosis, osteoarthritis or the formation of malignant tissue in the body. These negative feelings can spread to influence every aspect of our lives, destroying any chances that we may have of experiencing and appreciating true happiness and joy.

We can lift an immense burden of distress from our bodies and our minds if we are able to take back the power that we have in our lives and stop seeing ourselves as victims and to find the healing that comes from forgiveness. Therapies such as kinesiology or counselling or group-based personal growth work can help do this.

Counting our blessings, having an attitude of gratitude for the things that are good in our lives is a huge help towards good health! As an instance, we could consider the things that most of us take for granted. If we have two eyes, two arms and two legs that work, then we immediately have more than many others who struggle with impaired vision and/or mobility problems every day of their lives.

When we take a different view of life, we change our experience of it.

The power of seeing the world
without constant anxiety

When we walk around in a state of constant anxiety or we suffer from panic attacks, we often have no idea what the underlying factors may be. When asked what provokes or initiates their panic attacks, many people will say that they don't know. They recognise that they feel unsafe but the circumstances in which that occurs may appear to be random.

Others relate feelings of panic in well-defined situations (being in crowds, for example) or that their panic attacks started occurring following a specific incident or time in their lives.

Some may say that their nerves are always 'on edge' or that they are a "What if…?" person, repeatedly looking for possible problems and difficulties and hardly knowing what it is like to be calm and tranquil.

If relationships with others, whether at school/work/home or elsewhere in our lives, always seem to bring conflict and pain rather than love and support, then expectations of more-of-the-same gradually build up, leading to constant feelings of apprehension, mistrust and anxiety. If our world seems like an unsafe place for any reason, then we can become constantly anxious.

The pituitary gland in the brain, meanwhile, may be taking the physical impact of the stress. Sometimes called the 'master gland', it is responsible for sending out chemical messages (hormones) that help control our growth, blood pressure, metabolism, water balance in the body, thyroid function and the production of other hormones such as oestrogen and progesterone. The pituitary also controls the production of adrenalin, the hormone needed when we are under stress in order to ensure that we have energy to deal with the situation that is causing the stress. The effects of stress upon the physical body are many and varied and long-term stress can age the physical body considerably.

In addition, function of the spinal cord may also be negatively impacted by emotional stress and so the functions of our reflexes and central nervous system may be compromised too.

The power of seeing the world without constant fear

When fear rules our lives, it limits what we can achieve and accomplish. We may be constantly afraid that the stability of our lives will be threatened in some way or that our partner will leave us and we will be alone, or that our home or finances will be in peril and we will not have "enough".

We may run away from new opportunities that life offers us because of fear of failure. The possibility of judgement, or of rejection or negative reactions from others, can stop us living the life we want. We may be terrified that life will run out of our control completely.

The role of the kidneys includes filtering out waste products from the bloodstream into the urine ready for excretion from the body. The kidneys are also responsible for maintaining appropriate fluid levels in the body, helping to control blood pressure and calcium levels and stimulating the production of red blood cells in the bone marrow. Kidney problems are not always obvious and are often only diagnosed in regular health checks.

The kidneys bear the physical impact of constant fear and may become dysfunctional under the strain. Since the kidney meridian (energy pathway) is also linked to the health of eyes and ears, chronic levels of fear may also eventually contribute to eyesight and/or hearing problems. From a psychological viewpoint, those who "don't want to see" and/or "don't want to hear" may have underlying fears (perhaps fear of change or fear of failure, for example) that are ruling the decisions and choices that they make for themselves in life.

Kidneys also represent the base energy in our lives and so, if we live in constant fear, we drain the base energy, leading to a state of indecision (lack of interest in making a decision) and general lassitude. Kidney stones may be seen to indicate that the structure (values, beliefs, hopes, career, etc. etc.) on which you base your life may be ready for a review. In other words, have you made the best choices and decisions for yourself along the way? Or, if these choices and decisions were right at the time, are they still right for you now or do you need some changes to make them more relevant to your life from this point on?

The power of seeing the world without anguish

For those of us who have been diagnosed with a heart condition or who have problems with discs in the spine in the low back, it is possible that the agony of constant anguish is taking its toll on the physical body. The overpowering pain of bereavement with the passing of a loved one can leave us feeling totally unable to move forward in our lives. After losing someone dear to us, we may be unable to let them go on non-physical levels.

Continuing heartache from bereavement and loss may contribute to the symptoms of heart disease and/or low back pain. The grief that we carry (sometimes for years) can affect the lungs. A persistent cough that does not respond to treatment may be indicative of unresolved grief.

Graham had had chronic debilitating pain in his low back for many months and, as a consequence, he was sleeping in a chair at night because he could not lie down. Even small movements were causing him to wince in pain. His GP had prescribed painkillers and anti-inflammatory medication but these had not been able to keep him comfortable. Graham had been referred to an orthopaedic surgeon and was now on a waiting list for surgery on his lumbar spine.

In order to show just how badly his ability to move had been compromised, Graham attempted to bend forwards (as if to touch his toes) but cried out in pain as soon as he started moving forward from the vertical position and was unable to bend any further. In testing the area of pain using kinesiology, a link to "sibling" was indicated. I asked Graham whether he had any siblings. He replied that his only sibling, a brother, had passed away after struggling for many months with lung cancer. The two had always been close and Graham was very emotional as he told the story of his brother's illness.

I asked him how long it had been since the death of his brother. Graham replied "Sixteen months". I asked him how long he had been suffering with his own unrelenting back pain. Again, he replied "Sixteen months". The agony of his loss, compounded by feelings of helplessness at the suffering that he had witnessed in the last months of his brother's life as he had battled with cancer, had taken its toll on the discs in Graham's lumbar spine. Graham needed help in dealing with his emotions and moving on with his life following his bereavement. Further testing with kinesiology indicated the presence of toxic metal (mercury) trapped at the point of pain in his back.

After using kinesiology techniques to relieve his stress on emotional and mental levels, and taking appropriate nutritional supplements to help him excrete the toxic metal from his body, Graham was able to bend forwards and touch his toes!

There may be times when some specific situation in our life seems to be both irreversible and endless and is causing us to feel overpowered, helpless and trapped. We may feel as if there will never be any solution. If we can't see any "light at the end of the tunnel", the stress that we are under may be burdening the lymphatic system, contributing to symptoms of congestion, typically in the neck, the groin area, under the arms and/or swollen ankles. The lymph delivers nutrients to the cellular tissues and returns waste products from them to the eliminatory systems. The lymph nodes play an important part in the body's defence mechanisms. Immune function may be impaired when the ability of the lymphatic system to do its job effectively is compromised.

The power of seeing the world with good self-esteem

Life may seem to be demanding too much from us at times. If this becomes a permanent state and not just a temporary one, we may constantly feel totally inadequate, that we just can't cope or that we have extremes of responsibility that are just too much for us to handle. Maybe we feel that life isn't "sweet enough" on many levels and we crave sweet foods for comfort.

Eating a lot of sweet sugary foods places a heavy burden upon the pancreas. The pancreas produces insulin to help control blood sugar levels, as well as enzymes to help in the breakdown of foods in the gastrointestinal tract. When the pancreas is unable to do its job efficiently, poor digestion and mood swings may result and the risk of diabetes is raised.

We all know how eating a diet of sugary and processed foods can lead to excess weight. In this chapter, we are looking at the emotional factors affecting our health and so we need to ask ourselves why we continue to eat these foods that contribute nothing to our well-being. Sugar can be very addictive. The need for comfort can be a very strong driving force in our lives if we are feeling neglected, unloved, abandoned, lonely, isolated, depressed or unable to accept the loss of a loved one.

We may try to numb ourselves to traumatic memories or experiences by seeking comfort in excessive food or alcohol. When we are in need of constant comfort, we are in need of help to find resolution of the on-going pain and move on with our lives. This help could be in the form of counselling, kinesiology or group-based personal growth work and/or appropriate vibrational remedies (such as flower essences) to enable us to come to terms with our situation and move forward with a positive attitude and with purpose. Nutritional advice to change the diet to more nutrient-rich foods will also improve energy levels and help with motivation.

The power of seeing the world with good self-worth

We may not be aware that we have low self-worth until someone points out that we are always putting ourselves down. When we think that "There will never be anyone who loves me for me" or that we will always feel that we "aren't good enough" or believe that we don't deserve good things in our lives, then our low expectations become evident in many ways. We repeatedly manifest situations in which these same patterns show up as wrecked relationships and missed opportunities.

We constantly search for love and approval from others because we are unable to give it to ourselves. When self-hatred exists, it can result in deep feelings of unworthiness. These may, in turn, contribute to the manifestation of addictions to substances and/or patterns of behaviour (obsessive compulsive disorder, for example).

Many of us have issues with our siblings, perhaps now or in the past, or they may be on-going. If our relationships with our siblings are/were not good, then we may have always felt that we were compared unfavourably with them or that we lived in their shadow. We may have been separated from our siblings early in life or perhaps we were unaware that we had siblings. Whatever the issues may still be, is there any way that we might find some resolution, alleviate distress and bring peace to the situation? If the trauma that it brought has been buried or it remains unaddressed, it may contribute to sinus problems, neck and/or shoulder pain, problems with the left eye and/or allergies of all kinds.

Anne had presented with recurring neck and shoulder pain and neuralgia that had not responded to any treatment. She had had a course of physiotherapy as well as anti-inflammatory medication from her doctor. Anne's dentist had thoroughly checked her teeth and gums and could find no reason for her pain.

During her session, kinesiology testing showed that an event of major significance had occurred in Anne's life six years earlier. When I asked her what had occurred at that time, she replied that her only sibling, a sister, had died. She had had cancer. Anne's energy was indicating a "What about me?" situation in the symptom picture and Anne said "My sister was always my mother's favourite, and she still is. Even though she has now passed away, my mother still doesn't seem to notice me."

The blows to Anne's self-worth throughout her life from the constant poor comparison to her sister had reinforced her feelings of being invisible and unimportant and her neck, shoulders and jaw had illustrated the burden placed upon her body by the lack of any resolution. Through her kinesiology sessions, Anne was able to improve her relationship with her mother and let go of the feelings of sibling rivalry that she still carried even after the loss of her sister. She learned to truly value herself and to have the confidence to set up her own business serving her community, a long-held dream of hers that her new-found self-worth helped her manifest.

Molly had had a very painful shoulder problem for several years. Physiotherapy and anti-inflammatory medication had helped her to manage the pain but she was still limited in the use of the arm and shoulder and wanted to find the cause of the problem.

Kinesiology testing indicated that there were traces of toxic metal (mercury) present in the tissues of the shoulder. Molly had four amalgam fillings in her teeth and we discussed the possibility of working with a holistic dentist to remove the main source of the mercury and replace the dental amalgam with non-metallic materials. Molly was happy to do this and to take appropriate daily nutritional supplementation to support the dental work and to help the efficient excretion of the metal from her body.

Further kinesiology testing to determine what factors had allowed the metal to deposit in the tissues of her shoulder revealed a link to sibling issues. Molly had an older brother and their relationship was termed "stormy" by Molly. Kinesiology techniques helpful in addressing emotional conflict were used to reduce the stress in her system and Molly said that she felt confident in proposing that they meet to have a discussion on the issues that had divided them for so long and to move forward together in a mutually supportive relationship. Testing still showed more sibling issues, however, and I asked Molly whether she had any other siblings. She said there were none but she had always wanted a sister.

Arriving for her next appointment, Molly said that she had asked her mother whether she had ever lost a child and she had said that she had indeed lost a child, a girl, when Molly was two years old. Molly had in fact lost a sibling and, although she had never been told about it, her energy system indicated a situation of bereavement that needed healing. After using the appropriate kinesiology techniques to address the previously hidden grief, the shoulder pain disappeared completely.

These are just some examples of health problems and the issues that may be contributing to them from the emotional and mental levels of our being. We may be aware that we are not coping well with some part of our life but feel unable to do anything about it. We may not realise that our body is crying for help on a non-physical level when it shows us that it is struggling to function in some way. Whatever our physical symptoms are, there will be deep unresolved emotional and/or mental issues associated with the part, or parts, of the body that are linked to the symptoms.

These issues may have resulted from:

- Relationship problems
- Lack of self-worth and self-esteem
- Family breakdown and separation from loved ones
- Regret and remorse
- Resentment and bitterness
- Grief, loss and bereavement
- Resistance to change
- Breakdown of community in our towns and cities
- Inflexibility and rigidity of attitude
- Lack of acknowledgement for our achievements
- Change of circumstances (for example, in our finances or our jobs)
- Conflict and discord
- Beliefs and attitudes that are limiting our life
- Intolerance, impatience and frustration
- Disappointments and dashed expectations
- And, perhaps, not counting our blessings -- failing to look at what we DO have rather than what we don't.

Have you ever asked yourself:

- How much do I express my true self in my life? Am I living a life that makes my heart sing?
- Do I typically blame others for my problems and grumble that life isn't fair?
- Do I allow others to emotionally manipulate me in order to avoid having meaningful discussion about difficult issues?
- Do I hold back from expressing my true thoughts and feelings for fear of not being loved?

- Do I repeatedly focus on events that occurred earlier in my life that I cannot now "fix"?
- Do I seek to learn from past events in order to move forward with clarity and purpose?
- Do I live with heart? That is to say, do I show compassion and empathy for the plight of others and the world around me? Do I take time to compliment others on their successes, however big or small? Do I truly appreciate this planet, the natural world and all that life gives us?
- Do I have purpose and meaning in my life? Do I think of each new day as an opportunity to grow and learn and make the world a better place?

We make choices every day about how we conduct our lives. We decide what we will eat, how we will react to the emotional stresses of life and what attitudes we will adopt towards the situations in which we find ourselves.

We can address the problems of the body by considering the frequencies of the cells of its component parts. Life is a continuous cycle of change. There is movement within each cell of the body. As has been shown in quantum physics, everything is vibrating on its own individual frequency. The different types of tissue in every part of the body each have their own individual frequency. The frequency of lung tissue is different from that of pancreatic tissue, which is different from that of thyroid tissue, which is different from that of liver tissue, etc., etc.

Every emotion has a frequency. Every thought that you think and every feeling that you experience has its own frequency. The frequencies of thoughts and feelings affect the energy of the tissues in your body that have matching frequencies. Thus, constantly harbouring or suppressing negative thoughts and feelings may eventually result in detrimental effects upon the proper function of the corresponding organs, systems or glands.

So we need to find ways of dealing with our "stuff" if we want to be well. We can all help our body to function better if we can lift the burden that we relentlessly place upon it by persisting in carrying anger, guilt, rage, fear and our judgements about how life "should" be.

Our "stuff" has come from painful life experiences that have provided us with reasons to build unseen prisons for ourselves to protect us from further pain. These prisons feel like a place of safety that we need to have in order to hide us away from any further trauma that life may suddenly inflict upon us at any time. Inside them, our lives are run from a place of constantly trying to avoid more pain.

Our "stuff" can harden our hearts and minds and colour our whole experience of life's beauty and pleasures. We may constantly question the motives of others around us. We may persist in looking for possible problems all the time. We may make things more complicated than they need to be. We limit our lives and the expression of our true selves. We interpret life through the filter of our "stuff". In doing so, we can wreck our relationships, our happiness and our health.

Emotions govern the function of the autonomic nervous system which is responsible for the heartbeat, breathing, digestion and other activities within the body that we do not have to consciously think about or control. We have all at some time experienced rapid heartbeats or palpitations when we are highly stressed, or we may have been unable to breathe calmly in situations where we panic. There are other ways in which we can see that emotions do disturb the functions of the body, but it is important to remember that there are also many more ways that are not obvious to us. They occur deep within the body and have a long-term effect on our health rather than an immediate one.

The power of compassion

Sue was struggling with persistent low back pain on the right side as well as episodes of depression. She had a 3-year-old child and said she thought the pain was caused by carrying her child on her hip. Previous treatments of physiotherapy and a course of anti-inflammatory drugs had not provided any relief from the discomfort, even when she had stopped carrying the child.

Her first therapy session using kinesiology showed that the pain was associated with her relationship with her father. She immediately burst into tears and sobbed uncontrollably for some minutes. Amid the sobs, Sue voiced her rage at her father's actions and her feelings of isolation and hopelessness in a situation that she could not resolve.

Sue's father had left the family home when Sue was a young baby. Her mother was left to cope alone with an infant and two other young children. As Sue grew up, she was the only one of the three who had made any attempt to spend some time with their father and get to know him, but her approaches had always been met with a total lack of any response from him. She was left bewildered by his silence and had come to the conclusion that his only reason for refusing to have any contact with her must be that she was unlovable and, in some way, a "bad" person.

I asked Sue to consider another possibility in this situation. In acknowledging the truth that he had children, her father would be faced with some facts that he could not deny. The first was that he had deserted his partner and his three young children and he had offered no support whatsoever then or at any time since. The second fact was that he had not been fulfilling the role of a father in his children's lives. He had not been there to love them, protect them, guide them or ensure that their needs had been met. The third fact was that he had missed out on what could have been the greatest joy in his life: that of watching his children grow up.

Looking at ourselves in the mirror is not always easy. Sue told me that her father was an alcoholic and was numbing himself to life. She could now see that the truth was actually that he could not face himself and that to acknowledge her presence, and that of her two siblings, in his life would be a constant reminder of that. It became clear to her that he had taken what, to him, was the only way out when he denied her a place in his life. She now realised that her conclusion that she was unlovable and a "bad person" in his eyes could not be possible because he had never spent any time with any of his children since the day he had left the family home and he actually did not know her at all.

A month later, Sue told me that she had approached her father again with a very different perspective on their relationship and that he had now agreed to spend some time with her. And, in spite of continuing to carry her child on her hip, Sue now had no pain at all!

So it is evident that optimal health depends on "sorting our stuff"; that is to say that we must address the negativity we carry, rather than avoid it, deny it, ignore it, neglect it, exclude it, numb ourselves to it (via some kind of substance abuse, maybe) if we want to be well. Research in cellular biology has discovered that the biology of the body responds to thoughts and feelings, that the cells "listen" to the energy of thoughts and that the body, mind and immune system change with each emotional state.

Life is not ever going to seem fair. It is not going to seem fair to us since we are all working on different "stuff". That is to say, we are all unique and our talents, skills and difficulties in dealing with the challenges and opportunities that life brings to us are many and varied. Thus we cannot compare our own lives with that of others on any reasonable basis. The health problems that we experience can become our teachers. The physical body is showing us what our blocks are on other levels of our being.

We live in a toxic world. If we are happy and fulfilled, we do not get sick. The toxins in our environment typically gain entry to our bodies via the foods that we consume, the air that we breathe and the substances that we use on our skin. They come in (as inevitably they will) and they need to go out again promptly and completely if we are not to be affected by them. But when we carry negative emotions such as fear, anger, rage, guilt, etc., the toxins become trapped in the body and are not excreted as they should be. What we might call our "disappointments" to life's many challenges can stifle us and make us ill if we don't find appropriate ways to express them. In other words, carrying around feelings such as rage, bitterness or resentment can hugely increase our risk of health problems.

When we are negative about life, some or all of our routes of elimination for unwanted waste matter in the body (bowel, kidneys and lungs, for example) become dysfunctional. Thus the toxins are trapped in the body and we can't get rid of them efficiently. We are now in trouble. More toxins continue to come in and pile up on a daily basis, the body has to "park" them somewhere and the result is multiple problems in the way that it functions.

This way of looking at disease can account for someone who lives to a 'ripe old age' despite not taking care of his/her health in generally accepted ways. His/her positive attitude to life has made a huge contribution to his/her health and enabled the body to remove the rubbish effectively and slowed down the deterioration of the tissues.

We cannot compare the paths that our own lives take with those of others around us as we are all on different journeys, learning different lessons, facing different issues and dealing with them in our own unique way.

Consider also the ways in which our "stuff" contributes to ageing. Most of us are deeply unhappy about the ageing process and there is a saying "Inside every old person is a young one wondering what happened!" The wisdom we attain as we age is priceless, but we want to have it in a healthy body that is fit and capable of activity. Deterioration of the body can be alarming as the years advance and we dread infirmity and loss of our independence. So, if we can lift the burden of stress on the various parts of our system, imagine how much better they could function. And imagine what that could do for our lives in general!

CHAPTER 7

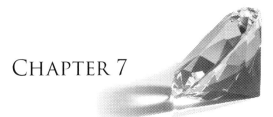

SAME THEME, DIFFERENT SCENERY.....

When you have a recurrent or on-going condition of poor health, your body is trying to show you what persistent pattern you are running that is damaging to you.

Throughout our lives, we are faced with repeated challenges and opportunities on physical, emotional and mental levels to show us what these patterns are. We have what can be called "same theme, different scenery". We find ourselves in situations that can teach us, but only if we are open to learning!

If we look at life as a school, then we can understand that we are being given lessons on an on-going basis. These lessons are woven into our daily lives in the shapes of our relationships with others and with the world around us. We are being shown our patterns of thinking, reacting and behaving.

If these patterns are not helpful to our wellbeing, then we are given more lessons of the same theme until we see the beliefs, expectations and fears that we hold that have contributed to difficult situations in our lives. We then have the choice of making a decision to change those attitudes and behaviours. If we do make appropriate and positive changes, then the lessons in that particular theme cease to occur.

If we refuse to acknowledge the lessons and continue to avoid facing the truth about them, we may eventually develop physical symptoms of some kind. When this happens, the physical body is trying to show us, via these symptoms, that there is a problem on another level that needs to be addressed. All too often, we allow ourselves to become physically very ill before we are willing to open our minds to the concept of dis-ease on other levels, not just the physical.

An example of this might be someone who always says yes to others when he/she needs to say no, one who repeatedly sacrifices his/her own wishes and goals in order to please others. When a person is unwilling to express his/her true thoughts and feelings for fear of negative reaction from others and the risk of not being loved by them, opportunities for self-development and personal growth are let go (travelling or working in another country, studying for a new career, or starting a new business, for instance). If suppression of the true self continues long-term, then the body starts to develop energetic patterns of restriction and limitation that may eventually lead to symptoms such as those of osteoarthritis, thyroid dysfunction and skin problems.

Imagine the physical, emotional and mental levels of health as a three-tier water cascade. When there is an unresolved problem at any of the levels, the water at that level becomes toxic. The physical is the bottom level of the three tiers (the "floor" upon which the other levels sit.). The emotional level sits directly above the physical. When we carry around negative emotions such as anger, rage, fear or guilt (to name just some of them), the water at that level becomes toxic and drips down onto the physical level, gradually corroding it over a period of time.

The third level of the cascade is the mental level where we hold our values, beliefs, attitudes, hopes, dreams, prejudices and expectations about life. Negativity at this level (for instance, a "poor me!" view of life, rebelling against its unfairness) results in toxic water dripping from this level down over the lower two levels, inflaming the emotions and adding to the corrosion of the "floor" (the physical level).

Thus the physical body (the "floor") is being repeatedly affected by issues occurring in the other two levels. These issues need to be addressed at the appropriate level; that is to say at their source. Treating the physical level in such a situation is treating the result of the problem and not the cause of it. Thus no long-term resolution is possible and the condition becomes on-going and chronic.

Looking at it another way, the walls of the unseen prison that you have built around yourself in order to avoid pain have been created from the experiences that you have accumulated on the mental level throughout your life. These constructs now shackle you to certain patterns of behaviour to protect you from the scary world outside. The walls come down and the shackles disappear when you see the patterns that are damaging you and you are willing and open to changing them. The emotions are then no longer inflamed and the physical body starts to heal itself as its struggle with the constant aggravation from the other levels ceases.

Brenda came to see me complaining of pain when passing urine. There had been some evidence of blood in her urine. She was 69 years old, an active playing member of a golf club and, in her words, feeling very fit for her age. She related a history of frequent urinary tract infections throughout her adult life and had been prescribed antibiotics for them each time they had occurred.

Brenda's doctor had recently ordered tests to be done on a sample of her urine and referred her to a consultant for further investigation. As a result of this, she had been given a diagnosis of a tumour in the bladder and had undergone surgery to remove it, followed by a course of chemotherapy over a period of six weeks. She was finding the shock of her current situation very difficult to handle and had got to the point when she had no interest in going out and, in any case, her bowel was now becoming a problem as well. Brenda was now visiting the toilet up to six times a day to empty her bowel urgently. In addition to the obvious inconvenience, this was a problem that she had never experienced before and added more fear to an already difficult situation for her.

Brenda did not really want to discuss her condition with anybody. Her husband told me that she refused to read any of the information given to her at the hospital and that she had told him to throw the leaflets away. She was firmly in denial but also in a lot of pain on more than just the physical level. In kinesiology sessions, Brenda's body took us to her teenage years to show us the patterns that were contributing to her physical problems.

During Brenda's childhood years, her father had been disabled as a result of a road traffic accident and was therefore very restricted in what he could physically do. He had been unable to take part in games or activities with the family and he had passed away in hospital following respiratory problems when Brenda was fifteen years old. Her mother had been diagnosed with breast cancer some months later and the trauma for the children seemed to be unending.

Brenda's sense of being totally out of control was understandably immense. And now it had come back once again, as if illuminated by some huge headlight focussed on her bladder. Her recurrent urinary tract infections had been pointing at the bladder as the common factor in her patterns of dis-ease for many years. In addition, the onset of bowel problems was now showing her that her body was urgently trying to rid itself of trauma from the past.

When I asked her how she had felt as a child with a home situation completely different to her schoolmates, she just shrugged her shoulders and said that it had been "okay". Instead of being with her friends, Brenda and her younger brother had had to help their mother with jobs around the house and garden that her father would normally have done if he had been well. Again, she insisted that it had been "okay". She had blocked her emotions then, just as she was doing now, in refusing to read the hospital information and refusing to talk about her feelings. Her body was showing her that she needed help in dealing with the trauma and that the deep emotional wounds from her teenage years were having a major effect on her health. Kinesiology provides methods of relieving emotional distress without the need for the person to discuss it and thus Brenda was able to gradually let go of the pain, reducing the aggravation of the tissues in bladder and bowel and aiding the healing process.

Stella was a 55-year-old lady, divorced and living alone. She had had lengthy episodes of depression throughout her adult life and had been prescribed a number of different anti-depressant drugs over the years, most of which she had refused to take.

Stella also had a bowel problem that had persisted through most of her life, despite trying everything that her doctors could offer. She had chronic constipation and had undergone a number of surgical procedures on the bowel that had not proved successful in resolving her problem. Since constipation shows that the rubbish of the past is not being removed effectively, it was clear that we needed to establish exactly what that rubbish was in her case.

Using kinesiology testing, the depression indicated a link to father-related issues and so I asked her about her relationship with him. Her father had ruled the home very strictly and had not ever shown any outward signs of affection to any of his children. He had developed health problems and passed away when his children were in their teenage years. Stella became very emotional when speaking of him ant it was clear that this subject was one that was still very painful for her.

Stella was silent for a minute or so, and then said that a family friend had repeatedly abused her through much of her childhood. She had been afraid to tell her strict and cold father as she had felt sure that she would be punished for fabricating stories. Her mother had never disagreed with his views and Stella felt that exposing the truth about what was happening to her would be greeted with disbelief and outrage that she had made such accusations about a long-term family friend. The man in question had long since passed away and Stella had remained silent about her trauma and decided that she had no option but to "get on with it" and pretend that it hadn't happened.

Of course, Stella's body was telling a different story. The poor bowel function that nothing had been able to relieve for so many years was a persistent demonstration that the suppressed trauma was having a huge negative effect on her life. Until she found a way of letting go of the intense pain of the memories, her bowel would not let go of the rubbish effectively. The experiences of her childhood with this man had wrecked her relationships with men over the years as the memories of the trauma were ever-present.

As we worked, over several sessions, with kinesiology techniques appropriate to situations of post-traumatic stress, Stella's bowel started to work more willingly and she experienced no further episodes of depression.

Dee suffered from debilitating pain in her back, legs and hips, pain in her ears, irritable bowel syndrome and she was overweight. Her energy levels were low and she was forcing herself to keep up a daily lifestyle of attending to the needs of others. She visited her elderly mother, did shopping for friends who were not mobile enough to do their own and dreamed of being well enough to use her creative talents in a business that she wanted to build with her sister.

As well as addressing the toxins trapped in her tissues and causing her physical discomfort, Dee's kinesiology sessions took us to times in her life at which she could recognise a common theme of suppressing her own hopes and dreams in order to support others in fulfilling their own ambitions. She said that she had never had time or the confidence to make herself the priority in her own life and that, if she had done so, she would have felt that it was somehow "bad", selfish and arrogant.

Dee was now at a point in her life when she lived alone, she owned her own house, and she now had the time and space in her life to devote to her hobbies. But Dee was in constant physical pain that restricted her activities.

She told me that she was waiting until she had fully regained her health before she would be prepared to contemplate the idea of setting up a business. She felt frustrated by the constant pain. She worried about cash-flow and was unclear about exactly what she wanted to do with her creative talents, with the result that she had consistent and permanent justification for delaying taking action to set up the business, and consequently prompting continual conflict with her sister.

We talked at length about looking at her situation the other way around. Instead of using her health problems as a reason for not fulfilling her dreams, how about looking at them as the result of not fulfilling her dreams? Frustration and blocked creativity can affect the ears and the meninges (the covering of the brain and spinal cord), and didn't Dee have symptoms that demonstrated this? And could the pain in her hips and legs not be showing her that she was blocking herself from moving forward on some level? Dee had undergone hip replacement surgery three years earlier.

Wasn't her body showing her that she was still holding the same beliefs and repeating the same behaviour patterns?

Dee looked excited at the possibility that she might actually improve her condition by expressing her true self in the work that she loved. However, this was swiftly followed by her protestations that her brain was" a muddle" and she felt so overwhelmed by the challenges of getting started that she had absolute justification in not doing it!

We talked about getting clear on her goals and on how she envisaged the proposed business would be a fit for them. She and her sister needed to draw up a plan of what would be required to get started in the business that they had talked about setting up for so long. As they got closer to making it a reality, Dee's pain reduced, her mobility increased and she was able to fully and happily engage in her new role.

Patsy presented with long-term irritable bowel syndrome that had not responded to the medications that she had tried over the years. She also had frequent sinusitis, and regularly used an inhaler for asthma. Her work required that she gave presentations to groups of people on a regular basis and the asthma and sinusitis often made this extremely difficult for her. When asked about her family relationships, Patsy said that she had been an only child. Her father and mother had divorced during Patsy's first year at school and she had remained with her mother. Her contact with her father had then reduced rapidly to nothing.

After several sessions and more bouts of sinusitis, it was clear that something was not being addressed adequately. Recurrent sinus problems can relate to distress in relationships with siblings, and Patsy had no siblings. Using kinesiology, trauma was indicated at a time in her life eleven years earlier. When I asked her what had happened at that age, Patsy burst into tears. It was the first time I had ever seen her express any emotion. She said that her father had passed away at that time, but that she had not attended his funeral because nobody had told her that he had died and she had learned of it a long time afterwards.

At this point, Patsy told the whole story for the first time. After leaving her mother, her father had eventually remarried and had more children with his second wife. Her stepmother had not wanted Patsy in their life at all and so her father had cut off all contact with his first daughter in sudden bewildering fashion for a child. She would have liked contact with her half-brother and half-sister and had recently discovered that her sister was living in a nearby town.

I asked Patsy what was preventing her from sending her sister a card or letter expressing how much she would like to see her. There was no answer to my question, just a look of amazement. It was a revelation to her that her sister might actually be pleased to see her too. And that a gentle approach to her might open up the possibility of being part of a whole new family that she yearned for. Sibling issues can affect the sinuses and wasn't it evident why the bouts of sinusitis had persisted? Grief can affect the lungs and wasn't the loss of her father and her siblings in her life being demonstrated in her asthma? And wasn't her bowel showing her that she was holding on to trauma from the past in some way?

Our thoughts, intentions, beliefs and expectations exist in energy form and affect the function of the invisible matrix that forms the human energy system. We have looked at the frequencies of emotions and how they affect the physical body in the previous chapter. Our thoughts, intentions, beliefs and expectations also have their own frequencies and affect the body in similar ways to emotions. Our cells respond to our perceptions of the outside world because these perceptions change our brain chemistry and our cells respond to that change. So our attitude to life is hugely important to our health.

If we are pessimistic or cynical, looking at life negatively, with a "glass half-empty" viewpoint, the tissues of our bodies that have frequencies similar to those of the negative thoughts will be correspondingly affected. An "attitude of gratitude" (that is to say, counting our blessings) is definitely good for our health and we need to be able to see the possibilities and opportunities that may be offered by the events that life brings to us, rather than the inconveniences.

Much of the stress in our modern lives centres around our issues with money, either directly or indirectly. This is a common theme, acquired in our childhood years, for most of us. We have beliefs such as "Money is the root of all evil" and "Money will always be scarce for people like me" and "If I had more money, I would be happy". Our hopes and dreams often involve having more money and so we view them as unachievable and impossible. As a result, the constant distress on the mental level drives us into patterns of living within a framework of constant lack, constant wanting and never having "enough". The aggravation to the emotions is unrelenting and they respond with anger, rage and/or fear. The physical body reacts to this continuing pressure by developing pain and inflammation, principally in the low back.

We may carry, consciously or subconsciously, negative beliefs about life, the universe and everything. Our life experiences reflect those beliefs back to us. For example, a belief that "Love always causes pain" will make us more likely to sabotage our relationships by constantly looking for problems in them that may result in pain. The resulting stress of each wrecked relationship then reinforces that particular belief and the cycle continues.

The outer state of our world reflects the inner state. Change must come from within to create a different experience of life.

Over time, the stresses that negative beliefs and expectations produce in our lives erode the ability of the immune system to do its job and they undermine proper function of the endocrine (hormonal) and respiratory systems. Thus some people may appear to age faster than others if their bodies are struggling, without any respite, under unrelenting burdens of negative beliefs and expectations.

We all accumulate "stuff" in our lives and, if we see it as opportunities to grow and learn, we can hold back the detrimental effects that are seen with advancing years. If we persist in blocking deep emotional wounds and mental scars and we refuse to get appropriate help to resolve them, the body will remind us, in bigger and harder lessons as the years advance, that the trauma is still there. We see more manifestations of "Same theme, different scenery".... The physical body will continue to reflect the non-physical levels of our energy system and show us, if we have persistent symptoms of dis-ease, that there are disturbances on other levels that are still not adequately addressed.

In this model of disease, a chronic condition may be viewed as an opportunity to change. In long-term conditions such as diabetes, heart disease, multiple sclerosis, etc., working at the non-physical levels helps the healing of the body and reduces the need to constantly manage the physical symptoms. If we only treat the physical level, are we doing the equivalent of washing the floor while something or someone is throwing buckets of mud onto it? And, if this is so, would it be more helpful to investigate the source of the buckets of mud rather than to only keep washing the floor?

CHAPTER 8

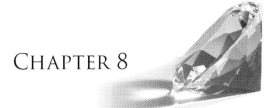

LIFE IS A CONSTANT PROCESS OF CHANGE

The human energy system is a complex field of intelligence that is invisible to our physical eyes. Light travels in waves and is measured in terms of its wavelength. Each shade of each colour has its own wavelength and so the wavelengths of the many shades of blue light are different from the wavelengths of the shades of red light, for example.

What we think of as empty space around us is not actually empty space. Our human eyes can only see light that falls within a certain bandwidth (the wavelengths of the colours of the rainbow spectrum). But there are other waves travelling through this "empty space" that we cannot see because their wavelengths are outside of this range (for instance, X-rays, gamma rays, ultra violet light). The signals that beam pictures to your television screen or those from your computer to your wireless printer are examples of non-visible waves travelling through this "empty space".

So we live in a kind of "energy soup". We cannot live in this "energy soup" around us without being affected by it. And as this "empty space" is intensified with signals from more and more masts for mobile phones and more and more high-tech 'gadgets' to make our lives easier (or so we might think), there is a heavy price to pay long-term in our health.

The brain manages the physiological functions of the body by electrical signals to and from every part of the body every second of your life and so there is an electrical field around the body. This field can be disturbed by the presence of other electrical fields. Thus it follows that it may be negatively affected by influences such as

- Computers
- Fluorescent lights
- Mobile/cordless phones
- Wireless equipment
- Geopathic stress (negative earth energies underneath your home or place of work)
- Living and/or working near pylons
- Radio alarm clocks next to the bed
- Smart meter(s) installed in your home or place of work
- Microwave technology
- X-rays
- Long-haul flights and some airport security machines

In these days of mobile phones and wireless technology, we have become used to the idea that there are invisible waves around us all the time. We are all used to switching on our radios and tuning in to the waveband frequency that we want to listen to (such as Classic FM or Radio 2). But many of us are very resistant to the idea that the human energy matrix comprises far more than the physical body that we can see.

So if this "energy soup" that we live in can adversely affect our health, how can this happen?

Interrupting and/or deflecting the electrical signals that constantly emanate from the brain to and from the rest of the body will mean that the signals are not received correctly (or not received at all). So, if these signals are influenced by electromagnetic pollution around us, then "the captain is no longer in charge of the ship". In other words, the brain is not able to control body functions properly. As a consequence, things start to go wrong without the appropriate control systems operating correctly.

Imagine the brain as the bridge of a ship, with thousands of dials showing the current status of its circuits, components and substances (blood pressure, for example). Let's say that, in a healthy balanced system, all the dials should be steady at a "six o'clock" position.

But, because of the electromagnetic pollution in the environment and the mental, emotional and physical stresses on the body (such as heat/cold, driving the car in heavy traffic, financial worries, family problems, and on and on....), many of the dials on the bridge of the ship are at other positions (such as at a "ten o'clock" position, or a "three o'clock" position, perhaps), indicating too much or too little (excess or deficiency) of the item being monitored.

The captain of the ship is constantly trying to bring all the dials back to their healthy "six o'clock" position and this must be done in the body's order of priority.

The "engine room" of the body (including the departments of heart, lungs, liver and kidneys).must be kept working efficiently every second of your life and has no opportunity to take a break. Other departments have a "work and rest" schedule (the digestive system, for example, that only has to work when you have eaten a meal), though they still cause major disruption when they are not functioning optimally.

The captain of the ship can take energy from other circuits as necessary to keep the engine room going. Thus, if you have an argument with your partner after having a meal and your blood pressure and heart rate have increased from the stress, the meal will sit in your stomach undigested until the stress abates, as energy has been taken from the digestive system to support the systems directly affected by the stress.

The fact that some of the dials on the bridge of the ship are not at their healthy stable positions may indicate that there are toxins in the body affecting the functions of the items being monitored. Mercury (toxic metal) may be inhibiting proper function of one of the heart valves, for instance, or parasites may be affecting the function of the ileo-caecal valve (commonly called the ICV) in the gastrointestinal tract between small and large intestines. This valve should open to allow food residue to pass through from small to large intestine and then close to prevent any backflow. If your ICV is jammed in an open position (a common situation for many people), then you will be reabsorbing some of your food waste back into the small intestine (a process called autointoxication, literally "self-poisoning") and you will be toxic and tired. Dark circles under your eyes are frequently an indication of this.

Prolonged periods of stress contribute to prolonged periods of ill-health. Shock, separation from loved ones, long-term financial problems and emotional conflict all take their toll on the energy system and subsequently on the physical body.

The human body is designed to heal itself. For each of us, our body is the part of our energy matrix that we can see with our physical eyes, but it is not the whole or only part. Energy flows through pathways called meridians and we have the tools in the modalities of kinesiology, shiatsu and acupuncture to assess whether energy is flowing along the meridians or whether it is blocked. When a given pathway is blocked, the body will find "work-arounds" so that it can "keep the show on the road", so to speak. By the time we develop physical symptoms, the body has been trying to compensate for the energy blockages for a long time.

A symptom is a message from the body that all is not well on one or more levels. If we regularly attend to the needs of the energy system, we can help prevent the possibility of problems arising in the physical body before they actually manifest. Your health is your most precious possession. Look after it well. Each of us is biochemically individual and the source of information about each of us is within us. The body provides us with a way of accessing that information without invasive methods or expensive equipment.

Energy testing or 'muscle testing' as used in the modality of kinesiology allows us to determine the parts of the human energy system that are not working correctly. The tests are not done to check the strength of muscles but to determine whether energy is blocked or not along any of its pathways within the body. This test requires only light pressure to a muscle to check whether it "locks" under a minimal load applied to it.

When an energy pathway is found to be blocked, this way of testing can be further used to provide information on why the pathway is blocked (emotional stress of some kind, or perhaps toxic metal, for example). In addition, it can determine what type of correction is needed to resolve the problem for that particular individual. The correction required may be nutritional such as a food, vitamin, mineral, herb or homeopathic remedy. It may be a flower essence for an emotional problem. It may simply be holding or rubbing specific acupuncture points on the body to enable energy to flow again optimally along its pathways.

Energy testing at this level is an art and takes practice to perfect. Since we know that our energy fields are affected by our thoughts, feelings, intentions and expectations, we must be clear of "opinions" of any kind about the result when we do the test (so we must have "brain in neutral" about the outcome of the test, so to speak).

Back to the subject of the influences of our environment upon our health, and there is one more aspect to be considered. This aspect is called geopathic stress or negative earth energies. You may have noticed that you feel unwell or depressed or listless if you stay for any length of time in certain places (in a certain room of your house, for example), as if your life-force is being drained out of you. This feeling goes away when you leave that particular area and returns when you go back to it. Perhaps you don't sleep well at home, but you do when away from home. Or you may hear people remark that there seems to be a high rate of staff sickness and absenteeism in those who work in certain buildings.

Such buildings are sometimes referred to as "sick buildings". Much investigative work on this subject has been done over many years in Germany. The negative energies that are draining your energy in this place are in the earth underneath the building. Healing sick buildings is a service offered by practitioners who specialise in determining the exact locations and patterns of flow of these negative energies. They can then transmute the draining effect into positive energies that provide a more uplifting environment for the body.

We cannot sustain life in a closed container. Our energy systems interact with the energies around us to provide "fuel" to maintain our vital force and power the functionality of the body.

Sally was a grandmother whose daughter and 3-year-old granddaughter were living with her. As her daughter was working, Sally took care of her granddaughter most of the time. She said that the child was having nightmares and had not slept properly any night since they had moved into their current house and so Sally was spending most of each night trying to calm her granddaughter so that her daughter could get some sleep before going to work. I recommended that the house was checked for geopathic stress and, from the very first night that the negative earth energies had been corrected, everyone in the house slept peacefully and well.

CHAPTER 9

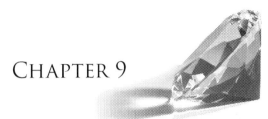

HOW CAN I HELP MYSELF?

If you want to lead a healthy life and reverse the damage to your cells, you need help in combatting the toxic environment in which you live (as discussed in chapter 5).

Of primary importance is your nutrition. The kind and quality of foods we eat is crucial for a healthy body -- it regenerates cells and tissues and is involved in the process of elimination. Without good nutrition, the body becomes toxic and deteriorates. Nature heals -- but it needs to be given the opportunity!

If your diet consists of processed foods, sugar, "fast foods", microwaved foods, trans-fats, then you will not be well. Your body needs adequate protein, vegetables and fruit (organic wherever possible). It does not need sugar, ice cream, cakes and puddings. Complex carbohydrates such as whole grains and root vegetables can provide the 'fill-factor'. Include green leafy vegetables as often as is possible. Protein, vitamins and minerals provide essential nutrients for the growth, maintenance and repair of our cells and tissues.

When cooking, use steaming, roasting or grilling rather than frying or microwaving where possible. Some people feel good on raw foods, others feel better on warm cooked foods. An appropriate diet containing both of these suits most people.

Commercial fizzy drinks may contain a lot of sugar and/or artificial sweeteners. They could be replaced by sparkling mineral water with a splash of apple juice to provide flavour. Black coffee or herbal teas (organic if possible) are more healthful than their milky counterparts. Eat fruit whole rather than in fruit juices so that you also have the fibre to help the passage of food residue through the colon.

Persistent pain in the low back may be indicative of dehydration. This is often a problem experienced by office workers who sit in the same position working at a desk for long periods of time and who do not drink enough water.

An irritable bowel will often happily tolerate foods made with spelt grain when it has difficulty with wheat (bread or pasta, for example). Skin problems and asthma are often reduced by removing cow's milk products from the diet. Goat's or sheep's milk products (cheese, yoghurt, etc.) are often a well-tolerated replacement. Joint pain may be reduced by eliminating foods containing sugar.

Our health is influenced by the ways in which our genes express themselves. We can protect our genes as much as possible by the choices we make about what we eat and drink, what we put on our skin (toiletries and cosmetics) and the environment that we live in (the effects of smoking, wi-fi, toxic household chemicals, for instance).

If you suffer from symptoms of hypoglycaemia (mood swings, headaches, shakiness, for example), you may find that you feel better when eating several small meals or healthy snacks daily rather than bigger meals after hours without food. Including some protein (poached or scrambled egg, for example) will help prevent fluctuations in blood sugar levels through the day.

If you have (or have ever had) dental amalgam fillings in your teeth, you may find that eating foods containing corn and/or oats in any form may make some or all of your symptoms worse (and this may include gravies and sauces thickened with cornflour too.)

Potatoes can aggravate some sensitive digestive systems (though sweet potatoes rarely do). Neither potatoes nor rice provide a lot of fibre for the bowel and so are not often helpful to a bowel that tends to be sluggish.

If you suspect that eating certain foods may be provoking all or some of your symptoms, you may want to find a qualified kinesiologist to test you for offending foods and/or chemicals and to investigate what toxins may be contributing to your symptoms.

And don't forget your toiletries and cosmetics too; it is possible that your shower gel, toothpaste, shampoo or other such personal products that enter your system through your skin or gums can be aggravating factors to your health problems and they may also need to be included in intolerance testing.

If you think that your symptoms may be due to virus, candida and/or parasites in your system, a kinesiologist, naturopath, herbalist or nutritionist can advise you on appropriate natural remedies.

Make sure that the quality of the water that you drink and use for cooking is good. There are many water filter systems available, including whole house systems and filters that fit onto shower heads, so that you can ensure the best water supply for all your needs.

Proper nutrition is essential for healing and maintaining life and, if you want to take the stress off your body and turn back the clock, you must provide the nourishment your body needs to repair and renew itself appropriately. In these days of what might be termed "unnatural foods", genetically modified foods, sprayed and/or irradiated foods, we commonly need to supplement our dietary intake with vitamins and minerals and nutritional complexes designed to support the body in processes such as detoxification.

Most nutritional supplements need to be taken with food to ensure that they are properly broken down in the gastrointestinal tract. Homeopathic remedies are usually taken away from food. A supplement containing a blend of nutrients to support optimal liver function is a good place to start as it will help lift the burden of toxicity that the body is struggling with. A qualified naturopath or nutrition advisor can help you determine what supplements would be appropriate for you.

Look for signs of vitamin/mineral deficiency such as:

- Tongue and inner lips are bright red instead of pink
- Corners of mouth are cracked
- Skin scaling at edges of nose
- Nails are ridged, brittle or soft
- Receding gums that bleed easily on brushing
- Lifeless thin hair with tendency to dandruff
- Low vitality, apathy and listlessness
- Muscle weakness, cramps
- Slow healing of cuts and grazes
- Mouth ulcers
- Poor appetite
- Poor memory, depression
- Teeth and bone problems

Reduce your exposure to plastics, particularly in relation to foods and drinks, wherever possible. A chemical frequently found in the manufacture of plastics is Bisphenol-A used in the production of some plastic bottles and linings of cans. When in contact with foods and drinks, the chemical can leach into them and be ingested into the body where it acts as an endocrine disruptor, leading to hormonal imbalances. It attaches to oestrogen receptor sites and has been linked to:

- Altered immune function
- Elevated risk of obesity
- Enlargement of prostate
- Disruption of female menstrual cycle
- Heart disease
- Diabetes
- Behavioural changes
- Impaired brain function
- Poor sleep

Use a non-plastic coffee mug rather than a take-away cup and lid. Drink fresh filtered water, if available, rather than water from plastic bottles. If using a plastic water bottle, ensure that it is not exposed to extremes of temperature (such as left standing in a car in the sun). Store foods in glass containers rather than plastic. Avoid the use of plastic wrap for your foods. Eat fresh rather than canned foods where possible. Avoid canned drinks and buy sauces etc. in glass containers rather than plastic ones.

If any of your teeth have been filled using dental amalgam, you may want to consider having the fillings replaced by non-toxic dental materials. There are a number of dentists who specialise in the safe removal of the dental amalgam and they typically advertise their dental practice as "holistic" or "mercury-free". Throughout the whole period of time (weeks/months) that the dental work is being done, it is wise to be also working with a healthcare professional who can advise you on a daily nutritional program that supports the safe removal of toxic metals from the body.

If your stress levels are consistently high, and/or you have chronic or persistent infections, you are more likely to have constant inflammation and this can cause significant damage to cells. You may find relaxation CD's, mindfulness or meditation helps. A self-help technique called Emotional Stress Release, taught in kinesiology, is detailed below. Alternatively, you may want to seek help from a professional (a kinesiologist, counsellor or hypnotherapist, for example) to assist you in finding appropriate ways of managing the problematic situation(s) and reducing your stress.

It is important to take care of the spine. Nerve impingement can contribute to adrenal exhaustion by setting up a constant "fight or flight" state, resulting in fatigue and chronic tiredness. If you suffer from back, head or neck pain, and/or you are low in energy, you may want to consider some treatment (such as osteopathy, for example) to help you structurally.

If you have a chronic bowel problem, colon hydrotherapy can help to clean the bowel. In addition, you may need further help from oral herbal remedies such as psyllium or slippery elm. Inflammatory bowel problems such as proctitis or diverticulitis may benefit from daily doses of aloe vera juice taken orally. A naturopath or nutritionist can advise you on appropriate remedies and doses.

If you don't sleep well, check your room for electromagnetic fields (EMFs) that may be affecting you. Remove mobile and/or cordless phones from your bedroom. Turn off wi-fi and electrical equipment at the wall socket; don't just leave them on standby mode. And do you really need to have your emails and the internet constantly available to you on your phone wherever you go? Some companies offer hand-held meters to measure the levels of EMFs in your home and it is possible to hire these meters on a weekly basis to check the levels in your immediate environment.

If, after this, you still don't sleep or feel well, then it is worth getting the house checked for negative earth energies (geopathic stress) by a suitably qualified professional.

If your problem is your working environment and this is not under your control, there are a variety of devices available to help protect your body from negative electromagnetic fields. These include personal protectors in the form of wristbands that can be worn all the time.

Emotional stress release

This is a simple, yet extremely powerful, technique to relieve stress, anxiety, fear, etc. It is also useful when you can't sleep because your mind is racing or worrying about something. It can be used to calm you in a current situation, or to prepare for a future stressful event such as an exam or an interview or a visit to the dentist. It can even be used to make a past situation easier to bear by relieving the emotional trauma associated with it.

There are two points on the forehead called the right and left frontal eminences. They are directly above the pupils of the eyes, about halfway up the forehead. They are specifically related to the brain and stomach meridians (energy pathways) and stimulate the flow of blood to the front part of the brain (which is involved when contemplating the present and the future). The rear part of the brain is involved in storing the memories of the past.

When using this technique, ensure that the stressful situation to be addressed is not complex. If, for example, the problem is around a marital breakdown, there are many aspects that may need attention, e.g. being alone, financial difficulties, finding somewhere to live, child care and custody, etc. In such a case, each aspect must be treated separately.

1. Lightly touch the left frontal eminence using the tips of the index and middle fingers of the left hand. Do not press into the forehead.

2. Lightly touch the right frontal eminence using the tips of the index and middle fingers of the right hand. Again, do not press into the forehead.

3. If the stress has a history, i.e. it is an ongoing situation from the past, use the two fingertips of one hand on one of the frontal eminences and the thumb of the same hand on the other frontal eminence. Lightly contact the back of the head with the other hand (by cupping the hand around the back of the head) at the same time.

4. Concentrate on the stress while the contact is maintained. Sometimes the stress is relieved very quickly. At others, it may require some time.

5. Completion is indicated by a yawn or sigh, or you may find yourself thinking of something completely different!

Finding an end to headaches

Some types of headache are relieved by rubbing a point called GB31 on the gallbladder meridian. Stand with your hands hanging loosely by your sides and touch the outer side of your thigh with the tip of your middle finger to locate the point required. Do not straighten or open the hands to do this. It is important that your hands are hanging loosely. Locate this point on both legs (it may be very sore) and massage both points firmly and continuously for one minute.

Relieving neck discomfort

If your neck feels stiff or uncomfortable when you turn your head to one side, hold your head in that position while 'unfurling' the outer edge of the ear to the rear.

What this means is that if, say, your neck hurts when you turn your head towards the right side, then you would 'unfurl' or lightly tug flat the outer edge of the right ear while keeping your head turned as far as is possible towards the right. Work all along the entire outer edge of the ear several times until your neck feels more comfortable when you turn your head.

Pain relief

This technique can provide relief of pain in some circumstances, so may be worth trying if you need help.

With the tips of your index and middle fingers together on either your right or left hand, as you prefer, trace the path of the infinity symbol (like a figure 8 on its side) in the air just over the area of pain. The overall size of the figure 8 that you trace is the same as the size of the area affected. Hold the fingertips about an inch above the area while the tracing is done as many times as is necessary. Make sure that the path of the fingers is upwards through the centre of the figure. If lying down, then the direction of the path is towards the top of the head.

Another way of reducing stress-related pain can be touching the frontal eminences with the thumb and fingers of one hand (as described in the Emotional Stress Release technique above) and placing the other hand over the area of pain so that the hand is lightly resting on the area.

Links

Websites that may help you find a qualified practitioner in your area include (for the UK):

General Naturopathic Council   www.gncouncil.co.uk
Natural Nutrition Association   www.nna-uk.com
Systematic Kinesiology   www.systematic-kinesiology.co.uk

National Institute of Medical   www.nimh.org.uk
Herbalists

British Institute for Allergy and Environmental Therapy	www.allergy.co.uk
The Society of Homeopaths	http://homeopathy-soh.org
Association of Registered Colon Hydrotherapists	www.colonic-association.org
British Society for Mercury-Free Dentistry	www.mercuryfreedentistry.org.uk
Information on electromagnetic fields	www.powerwatch.org.uk

About the Author

The author is a naturopath, kinesiologist and nutrition adviser. Born into a family with chronic health issues, she has been on a lifelong search to understand the meaning of disease in our lives and the learning that it brings through opening us to the wisdom innate in all of us.

liveyoungerlivewiser@gmail.com

Printed in the United States
By Bookmasters